DIABETES BEYOND NUMBERS

A COMPLETE GUIDE TO UNDERSTANDING DIABETES MANAGEMENT

NUZHAT CHALISA MD, FACE

Diabetes Beyond Numbers

Copyright © 2020 by Nuzhat Chalisa

Cover by Andy Meaden

Typesetting & Formatting by Black Bee Media

ISBN: 978-1-7355909-0-5

(PRINTABLE WORK SHEETS)

I want to make sure you get as much value as possible from this book.

As a way of saying thank you, I am offering my readers a workbook with the following very useful worksheets.

DIABETES SURVIVAL GUIDE

<u>5 different worksheets including:</u>

Glucose monitoring sheet

Diabetes care plan

Pandemics survival tips

Insulin dose calculation based on carb and correction

<u>Bonus:</u>

Pearls for a healthy lifestyle from my upcoming *Lifestyle 21 Program*.

If you are interested, please go to the website below.

https://www.nuzhatchalisamd.com/book

Dedication

This book is dedicated to my father, Saifuddin Kisat, who loved us endlessly till the day he died from complications of diabetes, and my mother, Farzana Kisat, a woman of exceptional courage and kindness who has always been there to shower me with her blessings in every aspect of my life.

I dedicate this book also to my daughter, Farah; my son, Amaan; my husband, Aamir; my siblings Shabbir, Nazneen, Durdana, Durriya & Abbasali, and every other family member who has supported me in this endeavor. Your constant encouragement makes my heart full and my life whole.

Table of Contents

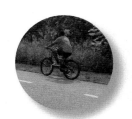

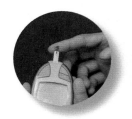

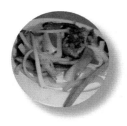

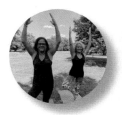

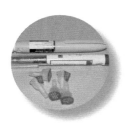

Types of Diabetes Medications
Oral Pills
Injectable Medications
Insulin Types
The Basal Bolus Regime
Injecting Insulin
Insulin Pumps

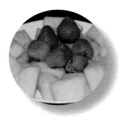

BMI
Goal Setting
Diet Diary
Tracking your Progress
Weight Loss Medication
Bariatric Surgery

Type of Diets: Which one is Better
Weight Loss Programs
Intermittent Fasting
How Fasting helps Lose Weight

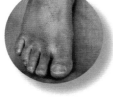

Acute Complications
Diabetic Ketoacidosis
Diabetic Non Ketotic Hyperosmolar State
Diabetes and Heart Disease & Stroke
How Diabetes affects Kidneys, Eyes and Feet
Diabetic Foot
Diabetic Gastroparesis
Psychological Problems with Diabetes
Diabetes Distress

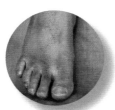
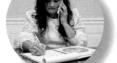
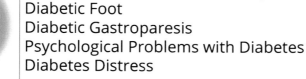

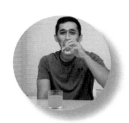
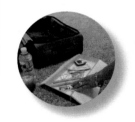
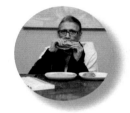
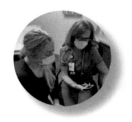

Today, diabetes has reached epidemic proportions. Over 415 million people in the world are living with diabetes which is about 1 in 11 adults. Forty-six percent of diabetics do not know they have diabetes, and the total number is expected to rise to 642 million by the year 2040. Doctors and patients have shared the struggle of diabetes management for quite some time. Almost everyone knows someone who is diabetic. Have our genes changed over time? Probably not. What has changed is our lifestyle. We eat out more often, stay at the office later, and are glued to technology instead of spending time outdoors. We've become less physically active, leading to more weight gain, which predisposes us to diabetes.

Until two decades ago, diabetes was a death sentence. People with diabetes were advised to completely restrict sugar, eat tasteless food, and take consistent insulin injections. Complications developed early on. Being a clinical endocrinologist and managing diabetes for over 20 years, I've seen the challenges a diabetic patient has to face over their lifetime. My passion to help people with diabetes was further ignited, fueled, and intensified after I lost my own father from diabetes complications, a few years back.

My father came to the United States in his early fifties to provide a bright future for his family. Like many other immigrants, he spent his early years working day and night to take care of us, and never gave enough time to taking care of himself. Luckily, aside from high blood pressure, he was fairly healthy—until about five years after his move, when he suffered a massive heart attack requiring three vessel coronary bypass surgery. He was also diagnosed with Type 2 diabetes around the same time. It is likely that he had diabetes long before he was diagnosed. His HbA1c at the time of diagnosis was over 13. Although he started to sporadically take medicine, he was still unable to afford continuous care for his diabetes or heart disease.

Five years later, he had another heart attack. The angiogram showed he had diffuse small vessel disease. This meant that smaller branches of his blood vessels supplying the heart were blocked, so despite his previous surgery to open his big coronary arteries, his heart was still not getting enough blood due to the blockade of smaller arteries. His kidney function also started to decline. By this time his kids, including myself, were older, his finances were stabilized, and he was finally able to get routine medical care.

For the next 10 years, he had several small vessel stents placed every 2-3 years. His diabetes was better controlled; he was taking insulin injections, since some of the injectable medications that are available now with protective effect on the heart were not available at that time. Over the next few years, his kidney function continued to worsen. He had persistent lower extremity cramps and pain due to peripheral vascular disease. His feet were getting numb due to neuropathy and his pulses were getting feeble due to blockage of small vessels in his feet.

He had progressive decline in kidney function and developed end stage renal disease requiring dialysis. He was started on dialysis 3 times a week. His heart disease had progressed significantly. He had developed heart failure and his heart function was only 15%. He was advised surgery, but he could not go for surgery until he had a defibrillator placed which would protect his heart from going into cardiac arrest.

While waiting to get the defibrillator his condition worsened, and the gangrene in his feet started spreading to his lower extremities. Doctors advised above knee amputation for both lower extremities. While I had seen this coming, it was a terrible shock for the rest of the family. He was admitted to the hospital for the surgery. He celebrated his 78th birthday with his family in the hospital while waiting for his surgery next morning. Sadly, before he could have his surgery, he developed sepsis and his heart failed. I could feel my heart sinking as I watched his pulse dropping with his head resting on my arms and his eyes looking at me saying, "save me please. I want to live." I wanted to save him, but it was too late. The years of uncontrolled diabetes and heart disease caught up to him and he was gone.

This is not an uncommon story. As a diabetes specialist, I have seen this tragedy repeated over and over again for patients with uncontrolled diabetes. Still, when I watched my own father die from complications of diabetes, my outlook on diabetes was forever changed. Knowing first-hand how finite life can be, I began to question my purpose and explore my passions. This led to the foundation of my nonprofit organization, Kisat Diabetes Organization, named after my father with the mission of creating awareness and providing education and early screening for diabetes complications.

The most heartbreaking part of my father's story is that he did not have to die like this. No one does. If diabetes is managed appropriately, these complications can be avoided. I share this story with you to show you how imperative it is to properly manage your diabetes, and how important it is to me to provide you with the right information to take care of diabetes in its early stages, before irreversible complications develop. With the right steps, the progression of your diabetes can slow down, and you can live a full, long, and happy life.

Today, we are fortunate to be in an era in which diabetes research has progressed exponentially in the last 15-20 years. We now know way more about diabetes than we ever did, and advancements in diabetes research and care have led to a better understanding of the pathophysiology of diabetes. New medications and technology, such as continuous glucose monitoring, insulin pumps, and various tools for diabetes education, have made it a more manageable disease. Additionally, our knowledge of how our diet affects diabetes has also changed. A diabetic does not have to cut back on sugar 100% and eat tasteless food. All you need is a balanced plate. With the implementation of these programs and technology, we may even be able to completely heal diabetes to a point where you have normal glucose levels, and prevent complications from developing altogether. Despite the challenges diabetes patients face, numerous opportunities to improve and protect your health are available.

The goal of this book is to help you identify and act upon these opportunities. This book is filled with a wealth of knowledge about diabetes, and written in layperson's terms without confusing medical jargon, so that any reader can understand the basics of diabetes better and feel more in control of their health. Reading this book will provide you with a clear understanding of what happens in diabetes, how it is related to heart disease and other medical problems, and why people develop diabetes complications. It will offer tips on various diet plans and information on new medications. Additionally, this book will provide you with advice on how to make the most of your doctor's appointments so that you can get maximum benefit from each visit. Ultimately, the book will help you to form a comprehensive game plan to manage and even heal your diabetes effectively. This book is for anyone who has diabetes, prediabetes, or a loved one with diabetes.

I have no doubt that this book will serve as your companion and guide in understanding and managing your diabetes. Do not be the person who misses out on an opportunity to take control of your health. Be someone who takes action immediately and take charge of your diabetes so that you can live a long, happy, and healthy life.

Chapter 1

UNDERSTANDING DIABETES

What is Diabetes?

Diabetes is a condition in which you have too much glucose in your blood because the body is not able to process glucose properly.

What is Glucose?

Glucose is the simplest form of sugar. Glucose is your body's main source of energy.

To understand diabetes, let us first understand how glucose is normally processed in our body. Glucose in our bodies comes from two sources: (1) the food we eat, and (2) our own glucose manufactured in the liver. When we eat, the carbohydrates in our food get broken into simple glucose. The glucose is then absorbed from the gut and goes into the bloodstream. From here, glucose has to enter the cells. To enter the cell, the glucose needs insulin.

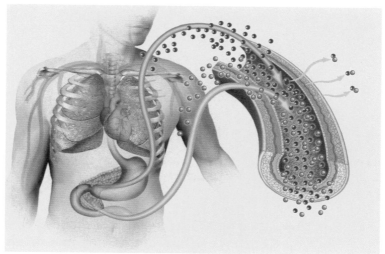

pancreas

What is Insulin?

Insulin is a hormone made by a gland called the pancreas. The pancreas releases insulin in response to eating. Insulin serves as the key that opens the cell doors, allowing glucose to enter. Without properly functioning insulin, glucose cannot enter the cell.

insulin allows glucose to enter

glucose can't enter cells

What Happens in Diabetes?

When you have Type 2 diabetes, the cells become resistant to the action of insulin so the glucose cannot enter into the cells. As a result, most of the glucose remains in the bloodstream, leading to high blood glucose. Since the insulin is not working properly, the pancreas works harder and harder to overcome the effect. As a result, after a while, the pancreas is burnt out and cannot make any more insulin. That is when people with Type 2 diabetes require insulin injections because medications that work through the pancreas are no longer effective.

pancreas can't make more insulin
injections needed

RISK FACTORS FOR DIABETES

Contrary to common misconception, diabetes is not caused by eating too much sugar. Development of diabetes involves a complex interaction between genetic, biological, and environmental factors. No test can show who would develop diabetes but certain risk factors increase your chances of developing diabetes, especially if you have the underlying predisposition. You may be at increased risk of diabetes if you are:

- Over the age of 45
- Overweight or obese
- Not physically active
- Have a family history of diabetes
- Asian American, African American, Hispanic, or Native American
- Have had gestational diabetes

Age: Your risk of diabetes increases with age. Therefore, it's recommended that everyone above age 45 should be screened for diabetes.

Weight: Your weight is an important risk factor for diabetes. People who are overweight and obese become insulin-resistant early on, which predisposes them to develop diabetes.

Race: Certain ethnic backgrounds have a higher risk of diabetes than others. For example, Native Americans, Hispanic, African Americans, and South Asians have a much higher risk of diabetes compared to Caucasians.

INSULIN RESISTANCE

Insulin resistance means that the body's cells are less sensitive to the action of insulin. Why does someone develop insulin resistance? Insulin resistance comes from a combination of their genetics and lifestyle. Many genetic factors predispose them to insulin resistance such as having a family history of diabetes and/or belonging to certain ethnic groups.

Women with polycystic ovarian syndrome (PCOS) also have insulin resistance. This is due to an excess of hormones, which opposes the actions of insulin. Because of this, women with PCOS are at a higher risk of diabetes.

Gestational diabetes is a form of diabetes that is diagnosed during pregnancy and goes away after pregnancy. Women with insulin resistance have a higher risk of developing gestational diabetes. Women who have gestational diabetes have increased risk of developing Type 2 diabetes down the road.

Sedentary lifestyle and lack of physical activity can also cause insulin resistance. During physical activity, muscles use up energy. When a person is not physically active, muscles become resistant to the action of insulin. Insulin resistance is directly proportional to the amount of body fat, specifically visceral fat.

The interesting part is that over 90 million people in the United States have insulin resistance, but not everyone with insulin resistance develops Type 2 diabetes. Why is that? This is because, under normal circumstances, the pancreas will work harder to make more insulin to overcome insulin resistance. This way, enough insulin action is available to keep glucose in a normal range. However, after a while, the pancreas starts giving up, and, consequently, glucose starts trending up. This is when a person develops prediabetes. If no intervention occurs, the process continues and the person develops diabetes.

Each individual's pancreas has a different capacity to fight insulin resistance.

Therefore, some people develop diabetes earlier than others. The development of diabetes also depends on if intervention is done early on. Increasing physical activity and losing weight can make cells more sensitive to insulin and prevent or delay progression to diabetes.

PREDIABETES

Prediabetes is a condition when your glucose level is above normal but not in a diabetic range. About a third of individuals in the United States have prediabetes. However, 90% of those with prediabetes are not aware they have it.

Why is it important to know if you are prediabetic? It turns out that by making appropriate changes in your lifestyle when in a prediabetic state you can delay or prevent diabetes completely. In 1996, the National Institutes of Health conducted a large study called the Diabetes Prevention Program (DPP). The purpose of this study was to see if lifestyle intervention with diet and exercise would delay or prevent the onset of diabetes in people who are at high risk for the disease. Results of the study showed that lifestyle intervention and metformin were very effective in decreasing the onset of diabetes. It was seen that by losing 5-7% body weight by lifestyle intervention decreases the risk of developing diabetes by 58%. This is by far the greatest amount of risk reduction seen compared to any diabetic drugs to date.

TYPE OF DIABETES

Diabetes is broadly classified into Type 1 and Type 2 diabetes.

Type 1 Diabetes

Type 1 diabetes accounts for 5% of all diabetes. It is autoimmune mediated, meaning the body's own cells called autoantibodies destroy the beta cells in the pancreas, resulting in complete insulin deficiency. Type 1 diabetes also used to be called juvenile diabetes because it is usually diagnosed at an early age. However, adults may also develop Type 1 diabetes.

Type 2 Diabetes

glucose wont enter cell

Type 2 diabetes, on the other hand, is caused by insulin resistance meaning the body is making insulin but it is not good quality and so, not allowing glucose to enter the cell. In Type 2 diabetes, some insulin is still working so there is a relative insulin deficiency. This type of diabetes can be treated with oral medications as well as with other injectable medications and insulin.

OTHER FORMS OF DIABETES

Gestational Diabetes

Gestational diabetes develops during pregnancy. It usually goes away after delivery of the baby. During pregnancy, several hormones are secreted that increase insulin resistance. For women who already have insulin resistance, it gets worse during pregnancy and leads to development of gestational diabetes. Gestational diabetes usually develops in the second trimester of pregnancy. Screening for gestational diabetes is done at 24-28 weeks with a glucose tolerance test. Gestational diabetes will be discussed in detail in a later section of the book.

LADA

Latent autoimmune diabetes in adults is an autoimmune diabetes that is a form of Type 1 diabetes but presents and behaves like Type 2 diabetes. It is therefore mistaken for Type 2 diabetes in many cases. LADA develops slowly over many years compared to classic Type 1 diabetes that develops quickly.

MODY

MODY stands for Maturity onset diabetes of the young. It is an uncommon form of Type 2 diabetes that is caused by a single gene defect. MODY behaves more like Type 1 diabetes. It affects young people with a family history of diabetes. This type of diabetes responds very well to oral medication and does not require insulin.

Secondary Diabetes

Diabetes can also occur as a result of other medical conditions and medications. Some conditions that can lead to diabetes are inflammation or surgical removal of the pancreas, pituitary or adrenal disorders, hemochromatosis, transplant surgery, infection, or malnutrition. Certain medications, such as steroids and immunosuppressive medications used in transplant patients, can also lead to diabetes.

METABOLIC SYNDROME

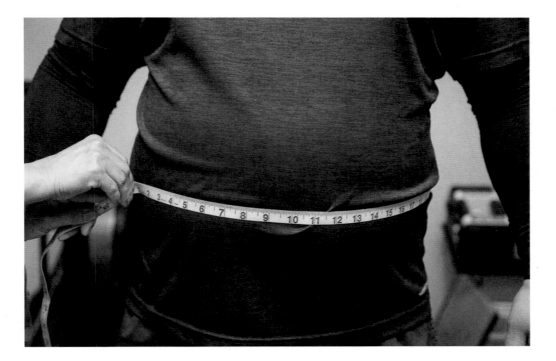

You may have heard the phrase "Metabolic Syndrome."

Metabolic Syndrome is a combination of metabolic disorders that render you prone to develop Type 2 diabetes, heart disease, and stroke. You may have metabolic syndrome if you have three or more of the following risk factors:

Table-1

Diagnostic criteria for Metabolic Syndrome Any 3 of 5 criteria constitute the categorical cut points Diagnosis of metabolic syndrome.	
Elevated waist circumference	> 102 cm or >40 inches in men > 88 cm or >35 inches in women
Elevated Triglycerides	> 150 mg/dl
HDL HDL	< 40 mg/dl in men < 50 mg/dl in women
BP	> 130 mm Hg systolic > 88 mm Hg diastolic
Fasting glucose	> 100 mm Hg

It is not clear whether Metabolic Syndrome has a single cause. It appears that it can be precipitated by multiple underlying risk factors. The two most important of these risk factors are abdominal obesity and insulin resistance. Metabolic syndrome is associated with a 5-fold increased risk for diabetes as compared with people without the syndrome

If you have Metabolic Syndrome, you must discuss it with your doctor. By taking appropriate measures to lose weight, increasing physical activity, and a eating a balanced diet, you can combat Metabolic Syndrome to prevent diabetes and certain other conditions.

Chapter 2

GLUCOSE MONITORING

DIAGNOSIS OF DIABETES

Now that you have a clear understanding of diabetes, let us see how you can find out if you have diabetes based on guidelines from the American Diabetes Association, the European Association for Study of Diabetes, and the International Diabetes Federation. Four tests can be used for diagnosis of diabetes. Not all four tests are needed for diagnosis. Usually if one test is abnormal, it is advisable to either repeat it on a different day or do a different test. However, if your doctor determines that your blood sugar is high, and if you have symptoms of diabetes, you may not need to repeat or do a second test. Diabetes can be diagnosed by HbA1c, fasting glucose levels, random glucose levels, or a 2-hour glucose tolerance test.

Hemoglobin A1c

HbA1c test, also called glycated hemoglobin, is a test that reflects your average glucose in the past 2-3 months. It measures the percentage of hemoglobin that is coated with glucose. Hemoglobin is the oxygen carrying protein in your blood. The higher the amount of glucose in the blood, the more will attach to hemoglobin. The higher your HbA1c level, the poorer your glucose control and the higher your risk of diabetes complications. There are certain conditions that can make HbA1c falsely high or low, in which case a different test may need to be done. Your doctor will be able to recognize these factors. For diagnosis of diabetes, HbA1c of less than 5.7 is considered normal. HbA1c between 5.7 to 6.4 is consistent with prediabetes, and HbA1c of 6.5 or above is consistent with diabetes. You do not need to fast for the HbA1c test.

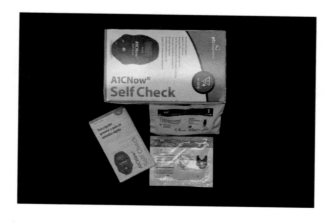

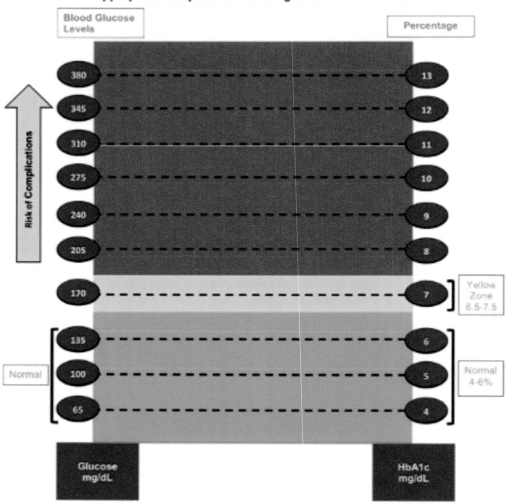

Appropriate comparison of blood glucose and A1c values

Fasting Glucose Test

Typically, your blood glucose level is lowest after an overnight fast. Fasting blood glucose is done after fasting overnight for about 8-10 hours. A fasting glucose level of 99 mg/dl or less is normal. A fasting glucose of 100-125 mg/dl is consistent with prediabetes, and a fasting glucose of 126 mg/dl and above is consistent with diabetes.

Random Glucose Test

Random glucose means glucose measured at any time of the day. A random glucose level of 200 or above is consistent with diabetes.

Glucose Tolerance Test

A glucose tolerance test is done by checking the patient's glucose level two hours after taking a 75-gram oral glucose load. A glucose level of 200 is consistent with diabetes. Due to the availability of more simple tests like fasting glucose and HbA1c, the glucose tolerance test is not usually used for diagnosis of diabetes. This test is routinely used to diagnose Gestational Diabetes.

Table-2

Diagnostic Criteria for Diabetes and Prediabetes Based on ADA Guidelines			
TEST	NORMAL	PREDIABETES	DIABETES
HbA1c	5.6 or less	5.7-6.4	6.5 or higher
Fasting Glucose Test	99 or less	100-125	126 or higher
Random Glucose Test	199 or less		200 or higher
2-Hour Glucose Tolerance Test	140 or less	140-199	200 or higher

SIGNS AND SYMPTOMS OF DIABETES

Type 2 diabetes does not have any signs and/or symptoms in its early stages. Lack of symptoms is one of the most important reasons why Type 2 diabetes remains undiagnosed in numerous individuals for many years. By the time the symptoms develop, diabetes is usually in an uncontrolled range and the patient may even have developed complications. Some of the warning signs and symptoms of Type 2 diabetes are:

- Polyuria (increased frequency of urination)
- Polydipsia (increased thirst)
- Polyphagia (increased appetite or constant hunger)
- Flu like symptoms
- Weakness or fatigue
- Blurred vision
- Slow healing of wounds
- Tingling and numbness in the feet
- Recurrent bladder infection
- Gum infections

MANAGEMENT OF DIABETES

Diabetes management or care plan refers to how you take care of diabetes and what your long-term goals are. Diabetes management essentially involves:

- Diabetes self-management
- Building a healthcare team
- Building a support system

Diabetes Self-Management

Self-management is by far the most important part of diabetes management. You are in charge of your diabetes. Controlling your blood glucose is the single most important goal to make you feel better and prevent long-term complications. Monitoring your blood glucose regularly is crucial in diabetes management. Keep track of your readings so that you can see how different types of food and different activities impact your glucose. Sharing your glucose numbers with your healthcare team will help them determine what kind of medications are most suitable for you and how well your current medications are working. It will also be a useful tool for your health care provider to adjust the medication doses and to see if you have any hyperglycemic or hypoglycemic excursions.

How Often Should You Test

How frequently one should check blood glucose levels varies from person to person depending on how well-controlled your diabetes is and what medications you are taking.

Individuals who have uncontrolled diabetes and those who are on a multiple-dose insulin regimen may have to test much more frequently compared to those on oral medications and other injectable medications who are relatively well controlled. Typically, for uncontrolled diabetes, it is recommended to check before meals and two hours after meals. In most other cases, it is recommended to check before each meal and bedtime. If you are on oral medications and have well-controlled diabetes, checking twice a day might be enough.

Additionally, you should also be checking glucose if there is a change in routine, like sudden plans to walk or exercise, a delayed meal, or if you are having symptoms of low blood glucose. You should check your glucose more frequently if you are sick or recovering from an illness or if you are on antibiotics or steroid medications, as these medications may increase or decrease blood glucose levels. People who take epidural and other steroid injections for chronic pain and/or other reasons may have to monitor glucose frequently after taking the injection, as the injections will significantly raise blood glucose levels and the effects may last for up to three to four weeks. Target glucose goals for blood glucose also vary from person to person, depending on the age of the person, controlled nature of the diabetes, and presence of complications or comorbidities.

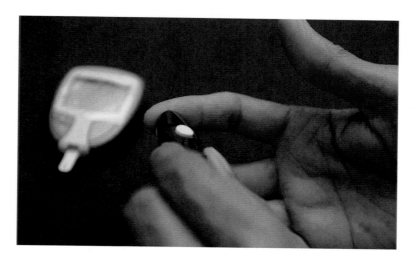

Based on ADA guidelines, it is recommended that pre-meal glucose should be between 80 and 130 mg/dl and two hours post-meal glucose should be less than 180 mg/dl. Glucose goals can be tighter or less stringent in some cases. For example, in a younger person without any complications or comorbidities, the glucose goal is stricter for tighter control of diabetes and preventing complications. On the other hand, an elderly person with comorbidities like heart disease, renal failure and hypoglycemia may need a much less stringent goal. Exactly what is an appropriate target glucose for you is a discussion you must have with your healthcare team.

Choosing a Glucose Monitor

Several different glucose monitors are available. Each monitor uses specific kinds of strips and has an expiration date. Some monitors may require charging while others are battery operated. You must do some research before you buy a glucose monitor. Sometimes, your doctor's office might be able to give you a glucose monitor free of cost; however, you will still need to buy the test strips. Before you invest in a meter, you must find out the cost of the strips and insurance coverage if applicable, to make sure it is affordable for long-term use.

Special meters are available with a bigger screen and display for people with poor vision. Also available are special glucose monitors called the talking meters for those who are legally blind. Meters have settings for pre-meal and post-meal glucose. Try to learn your meter and adjust those settings based on your meal times. Some meters have the capability of downloading the information, which you can then print out and take to your doctor's office.

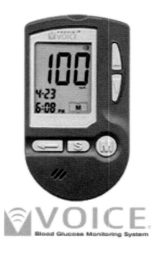

Most meters will only take one to two minutes to check the glucose; others will give you the results within a few seconds.

How to Use the Glucose Meter

Before using a glucose meter, you must wash your hands with soap and water. An alcohol swab may be used, however, the hands must be dried completely after using the alcohol swab, as the alcohol might interfere with the blood glucose reading. Using a glucose meter is a very easy process and takes only a couple of minutes.

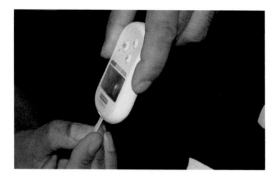

- Most meters have a lancet device that you can use to prick your finger
- Insert the needle in the lancet device

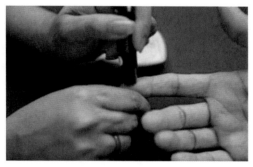

- Use the Lancet to prick your finger

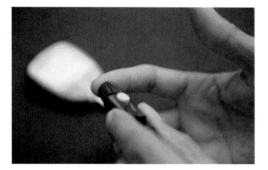

- Gently squeeze your finger to bring a small drop of blood. It's advisable to discard the first drop of blood and use the second drop of blood for testing
- Take the test strip close to the drop of blood. Most test strips have the capability to suck the blood in. Some may require putting the drop of blood on the test strips

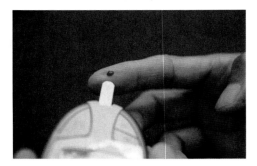

- Insert the test strips into the meter. The meter then displays your blood glucose reading. Some meters may require inserting the test strip first before you put the drop of blood on it
- Read the instructions carefully before you start testing
- Your reading is usually stored in the meter
- If you see unexpectedly high or low readings, wash your hands and test again
- Make sure the test strips are not expired

Alternate Site Testing

Some glucose meters are FDA approved to be tested on sites other than your fingertips, including your thighs, calf, upper arms, and forearms. Sites other than your fingers can only be used if your glucose is stable, as this may not be very accurate. You must check your glucose using fingertips if your glucose is lower or higher than expected.

Continuous Glucose Monitors (CGM)

A continuous glucose monitor is a device that attaches to your body to check glucose continuously throughout the day and night. Several different types of continuous glucose monitors are available and each has a specific sensor, a transmitter, and a receiver that displays and stores the readings. Continuous glucose monitors have the capability to download the glucose readings and trends, which can be printed for review. Continuous glucose monitors help you see how glucose levels are affected by certain types of foods and activities. They will also keep track of your glucose while you are sleeping, and keep a check for hyperglycemia or hypoglycemia.

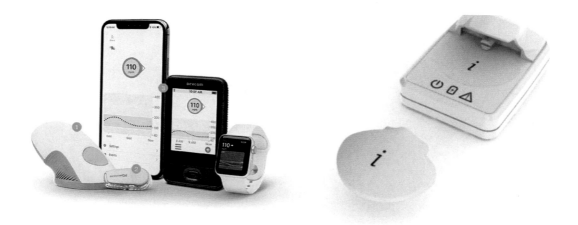

Continuous glucose monitors also have programmable alerts if your glucose is going too low or too high. Most people find CGM very helpful, since they allow patients to prevent pricking their fingers multiple times. Some of the commonly used continuous glucose monitors are Freestyle Libre, Dexcom, and Medtronic Guardian.

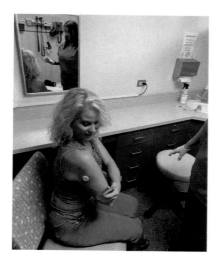

CGM like Freestyle Libre can be used by downloading an app on your smart phone, which then allows you to use your phone to scan your glucose on the sensor. Alternatively, continuous monitors like Dexcom work via Bluetooth and allow not only you, but also your loved one or your health care provider, to have access to your sensor information remotely. Continuous glucose monitors are becoming more popular and more insurance companies are providing coverage for them.

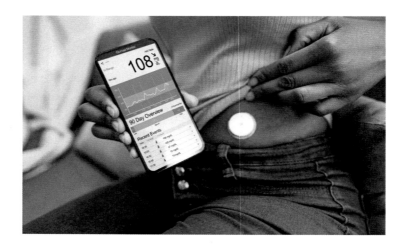

What to do with the High and Low values?

Persistently elevated blood glucose can lead to complications. If you check your glucose and it is unusually higher than normal, then you may need to take some action. First, ask yourself why your glucose reading is high. Perhaps you have had something in your meal that spiked up your glucose, or you may have had a snack after a meal? Did you forget to take your medications today? Are you sick, stressed, or in pain? Unfortunately, a single high glucose reading does not give you any symptoms. Talk to your doctor about how you want to manage the high glucose readings. In most cases, as long as the glucose is not very high, you may want to watch your diet and monitor closely for the next 24 hours. If high readings persist, you may want to call your doctor with the readings to get further instructions. If you are on insulin, your doctor might have given you instructions on taking extra insulin when your glucose is high.

If you already know you have had something in your meal that spiked up your glucose levels like a piece of cake or dessert, then you may want to just wait and be careful about what you are eating until your next meal. However, if your glucose is very high, usually over 400, you must call your provider and may need to go to the Emergency Room to get evaluated for diabetic ketoacidosis. Ketoacidosis will be discussed in detail in a later section.

Why Does my Blood Glucose Go High Even When I am Not Eating?

If you are a diabetic, you may have noticed higher glucose in the morning even if you have not eaten much the night before. There are several reasons for this. In addition to what you eat, your body also gets glucose from your liver. The liver can convert stored glycogen to glucose. Between meals and during fasting the liver continues to supply glucose to provide fuel for the body. Additionally, overnight, the body makes several hormones like cortisol and growth hormone that raise your blood glucose.

You should avoid skipping meals in trying to lower blood glucose, as skipping meals turns the body into the fasting mode and activates the liver to release glucose, which can lead to high glucose. Skipping meals can also lead to overeating, which can cause hyperglycemia and weight gain.

HYPOGLYCEMIA

Abnormally low blood glucose is called hypoglycemia. It is usually defined as glucose below 70; however, the cutoff for low glucose may vary in different individuals. You need to know what the low value is for you. You and your healthcare providers should discuss this number. If not treated correctly and promptly, hypoglycemia can be dangerous, especially if you are driving a vehicle. Severe hypoglycemia can lead to loss of consciousness, seizures, and coma. Hypoglycemia can occur in several situations. In most cases, there is an identifiable reason for it, and identifying this reason can help prevent future episodes of hypoglycemia.

Scenarios for Low Blood Glucose

- Delayed meal
- Skipping a meal
- Increased physical activity
- Taking too much insulin
- Certain medications like sulfonylureas can last in your body longer and cause hypoglycemia
- Medications like antibiotics can cause hypoglycemia when you are sick and not eating enough
- Drinking too much alcohol on an empty stomach

Signs and Symptoms of Hypoglycemia

- Dizziness
- Lightheadedness
- Sweating
- Shaking
- Confusion
- Irritability
- Weakness
- Hunger
- Sleepiness

- Tingling and numbness
- Blurred vision
- Seizures
- Loss of consciousness
- Coma

Hypoglycemic Unawareness

Some people with long-term uncontrolled diabetes may not feel the symptoms of hypoglycemia due to nerve damage. This is called a hypoglycemic unawareness. This can be really dangerous as you would not know you are hypoglycemic until it is severe enough to potentially cause loss of consciousness or seizure. The only way to keep a check is frequent monitoring. Use of continuous glucose monitors can be very useful and are highly recommended in this setting.

GLUCAGON

If hypoglycemia is not treated immediately, you may pass out and become unconscious. In this situation, you will need assistance by a family member or someone else to give you an injection of glucagon. Glucagon is a hormone that your pancreas makes to raise blood glucose. Glucagon can increase blood glucose within minutes of injecting. You must have a glucagon kit with you all the time if you are on diabetes medications, especially insulin. A glucagon kit has an injection that can be used by a friend or a caregiver in case you lose consciousness. It would be a good idea to teach some close friends and family members whom you usually spend time with so they can give you the injection if needed. Glucagon is now also available in powder form that has to be administered into the nostril via an intranasal device. Nasal glucagon is inserted into the nose but does not have to be inhaled. Once a person wakes up after taking glucagon, they must take a fast-acting source of sugar and then a small snack, as glucagon will only last in the system for a few minutes.

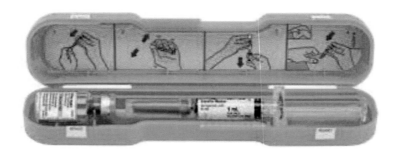

Treatment of Hypoglycemia

It is important to treat hypoglycemia right away. A good way is to use the 15 grams rule.

15 Grams Rule for Treatment of Hypoglycemia

According to the 15 grams rule, if you have low glucose, usually below 70 mg/dl, you treat it with 15 grams of fast acting sugar, then wait for 15 minutes and check your glucose again. If your glucose is still low, take another 15 grams of carbohydrate. This way, you will avoid overshooting, which leads to high glucose down the road.

Examples of Fast Acting Sugars That Can be Used to Treat Hypoglycemia

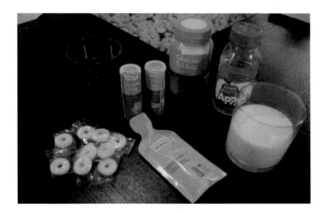

Examples of 15 grams of Glucose

- Glucose tablets, three glucose tablets (5 grams each)
- One tube of glucose gel
- 4-6 pieces of hard candy (not sugar-free)
- 4 ounces of fruit juice or soda (half cup)
- 2 tablespoons of raisins
- 1 cup skim milk
- 1 teaspoon table sugar
- 8-10 Life Savers

Sometimes, if your glucose has been running very high for a long time, when you start getting treated and your glucose starts coming down, you may have symptoms of hypoglycemia, even at a higher level of glucose, since your body is not used to the normal glucose levels and may perceive normal glucose as low. This should go away as your glucose levels start improving over time.

Chapter 3

DIABETES MANAGEMENT PLAN

DOCTOR VISITS

Most diabetes will be initially managed by a primary care physician. However, if your diabetes is not well-managed, you must be seen by a specialist, called an endocrinologist, for proper management of diabetes. Sometimes, a primary care physician who has many different issues to address may not have enough time to address diabetes management in depth. Therefore, seeing a specialist who would focus just on your diabetes is helpful.

Ideally, a reasonably well controlled diabetic needs to be seen every three months. If your glucose is high, your doctor may ask you to be seen sooner. To make the most out of your visit, it is important to make a list of information that you want to share or discuss with your doctor. Always take your glucose logs or any outside labs that your doctor does not have access to, and an updated medication list with you when you go for your appointment. Also, make a list of questions that you want to discuss with your doctor. Do not hesitate to ask questions. When you get started on a new medication, ask how it works, what to expect in the next couple of weeks, and if there are any side effects.

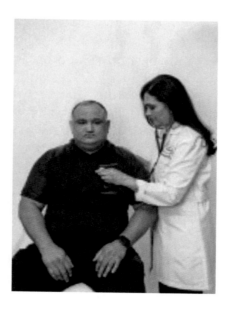

LABS

Some doctors may want to order labs in advance so you have results to discuss when you see them. Others will do labs on the day of the appointment. Talk to your doctor how they want to pursue your labs. Following are the tests and their frequency of testing based on The American Diabetes Association's recommendations. Some patients may need more frequent testing based on the presence of certain complications.

Table-3

LAB	FREQUENCY OF TESTING
Hga1c	Every 3 months
Creatinine	Once a year
Lipid panel	Once a year
Urine micro albumin	Once a year
Blood pressure	Every visit
Weight	Every visit
Eye exam	Once a year
Foot exam	Once a year

Hemoglobin A1c (HbA1C)

HbA1C, also called glycated hemoglobin, is a blood test that gives the average blood glucose over a period of the past three months. This test is a tool that gives you an overall idea of how well your diabetes is controlled. HbA1c levels must be checked every three months. HbA1c in most people must be maintained under 7.0. Once HbA1c increases above 7.0, the risk for developing complications from diabetes also increases. HbA1c goals may vary in certain individuals based on the person's age and the presence of complications. For example, it is very reasonable to have a HbA1c goal of 8.0 in an elderly frail person with increased risk of hypoglycemia. Similarly, HbA1c goal is also slightly higher in patients with severe cardiovascular complications or stroke, since hypoglycemia in these individuals may be more harmful than slightly elevated blood glucose.

Certain conditions can alter your HbA1c and give you a false high or false low result. For example, people with iron deficiency anaemia may have a false high HbA1c, whereas people with anaemia of chronic disease or renal failure may have a false low HbA1c. It is important to understand that HbA1c is based on your average glucose levels; therefore, if you are having frequent low and high glucose excursions, your HbA1c may look like normal. Or if you are having frequent hypoglycemic reactions, then your HbA1c may come lower despite having higher glucose the rest of the time.

Lipid Panel

A lipid panel measures the level of total good and bad cholesterol in your blood, which indicate your risk of having a heart attack. Since diabetes and heart disease are so closely related and people with diabetes have a much higher risk of having heart disease, monitoring lipids is a routine part of diabetes management. It is recommended to monitor your lipids at least once a year. Sometimes, if you are started on a cholesterol medication or your dose is changed, it may have to be checked sooner.

Lipid Goals for Diabetics Based on ADA Guidelines

Table-4

Total cholesterol	< 200
Triglycerides	< 150
LDL (Low density lipoprotein)	< 100
HDL (High density lipoprotein)	> 50

If your cholesterol is higher than the goal, you may have to be started on medication.

Statins

Statins are a class of medication that are used as a first-line agent for treatment of high cholesterol. Statins have many benefits. Multiple studies have shown that statins significantly decrease the risk of having a heart attack. Since diabetics have similar changes in their blood vessels as people with coronary artery disease, the American Diabetes Association recommends that all diabetic patients between 45 and 75 years of age must be on a statin medication even if their cholesterol is in normal range. The type of statin and the dose usually depend on the level of cholesterol and extent of cardiovascular disease risk.

RENAL FUNCTION

Since diabetes affects your kidneys, it is important that renal function be monitored periodically. Two tests are used to monitor renal functions: Serum creatinine and Urine micro albumin to creatinine ratio.

Serum Creatinine

Creatinine levels in the blood can provide your doctor with information about how well your kidneys are working. Creatinine is the waste product that forms when the protein creatine, which is found in your muscles, breaks down. Each kidney has millions of small filtering units called nephrons. The nephrons constantly filter blood through a very tiny cluster of blood vessels called glomeruli. These structures filter waste products, excess water, and other toxins out of the blood. Creatinine is one of the substances that the kidneys normally eliminates from the body. If the level of creatinine is higher than a certain range, it indicates kidney damage. Normal values of creatinine for a person may vary depending on age, sex, and racial background. Serum creatinine level must be checked at least once a year. If the creatinine is high, it should be monitored more frequently or your doctor may involve a kidney specialist.

Urine Microalbumin to Creatinine Ratio

The Urine microalbumin is a test that detects tiny amounts of protein in your urine. When your kidneys are functioning normally, they remove the waste products from the blood and keep the protein and other nutrients in the blood. However, when the kidneys are not functioning properly, they will not be able to keep the protein in the blood, so the protein starts leaking into the urine. The more severe the kidney damage, the more protein will leak into the urine. Urine micro-albumin tests checks if your kidneys are leaking small amounts of protein and helps to diagnose kidney damage in early stages.

Table-5

Microalbumin < 30	Normal
Microalbumin 30-300	Micro albuminuria (Early kidney damage)
Microalbumin >300	Macro albuminuria (Advanced kidney damage)

BLOOD PRESSURE

High blood pressure damages the blood vessels in the same way as diabetes. Therefore, having both diabetes and high blood pressure significantly increases the risk of having a heart attack or stroke. The American Diabetes Association recommends BP goal of less than 140/80 for diabetics. If BP is higher than goal, lifestyle modification with diet and exercise, weight loss, smoking cessation, and reduced salt and alcohol intake is advised.

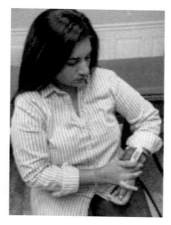

If BP is still high, blood pressure lowering medication is started. Certain medications work better in diabetics than others. A group of medications called ACE inhibitors (angiotensin converting enzyme inhibitors) or ARB (angiotensin receptor blockers) are usually advised to be used as first-line agents for BP control in diabetics. These medications, in addition to lowering BP, also have a protective effect on the kidneys.

EYE EXAM

The American Diabetes Association recommends a comprehensive eye exam for all diabetics upon diagnosis and then yearly or sooner if retinopathy is present.

Eye damage from diabetes does not cause any vision changes in early stages. By the time visual symptoms develop, retinopathy might be irreversible. Early retinopathy can be picked up on a routine eye exam and treated.

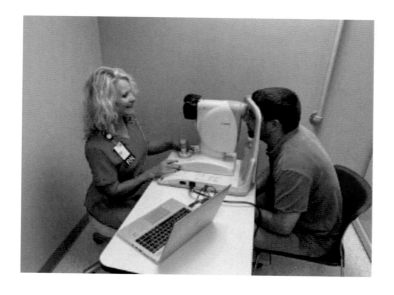

FOOT EXAM

As a diabetic, it is recommended that you have a foot exam by your health care provider at every visit and a comprehensive foot exam by a podiatrist once a year. Diabetics are prone to develop dry feet, callus, ingrown toenails, fungus in the nails, and other infections.

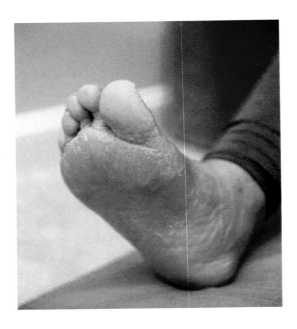

DIABETIC SELF-FOOT CARE

All diabetics must inspect their feet and care for them every day as follows:

- Look for cuts or breaks in the skin
- Look for swelling or ulcers
- Look in between the toes and keep the area dry
- Wash their feet every day
- Avoid wearing sandals or tight shoes
- Avoid walking barefoot
- Avoid using scissors, or knife to trim toe nails

Chapter 4

MANAGEMENT OF DIABETES

DIET MANAGEMENT

Lifestyle changes with behavior modification, healthy eating, and portion sizing is the key to the management of diabetes. Although there are some basic principles that apply to all kinds of diets, nutritional requirements in diabetics may vary from person to person. No generic nutrition plan works best for everyone. In other words, there is no such thing as a standard diabetic diet. Your diet will vary depending on what you are trying to achieve.

Before you start planning a diet, you must ask yourself the following questions:

1. What is your goal?
2. Are you overweight and trying to cut calories?
3. Is your diabetes well controlled?
4. Are you trying to adjust your diet to maintain your diabetes in good control?

Contrary to popular belief, having diabetes does not mean you have to give up on eating, start eating special foods, or follow complicated diet plans.

Healthy eating translates into upgrading your diet with small changes like making smart choices and portion sizing while enjoying nutrition and great taste. A diabetic diet is based on eating three meals a day with small healthy snacks in between meals if needed. This helps your body to use insulin more effectively.

Getting a registered dietitian or a diabetes educator involved can be very helpful to put together a diet plan based on your health goals, tastes, and lifestyle. A dietitian can also give useful suggestions on how to improve your eating habits such as portion sizing based on your own weight and activity levels. No matter what diet plan you adopt the basic principles of medical nutrition therapy in diabetes remains the same. The following are some basic concepts and principles that are adopted for a balanced diet. Each of these will be discussed in detail.

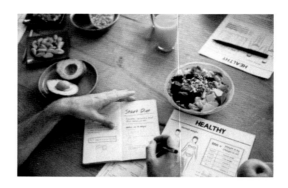

BASIC PRINCIPLES OF A DIABETIC DIET

- Creating a custom-made healthy eating plan for yourself
- Planning your meal
- Portion sizing
- Balancing your plate
- Having consistent meals at regular times
- Maintaining a healthy weight
- Limiting use of sweetened beverages
- Limiting use of alcohol
- Reading nutrition labels
- Carbohydrate counting
- Keeping a check on the total calories you take in

Before we indulge into the nitty gritty of diet management, it is important to get some basic information about different types of nutrients.

TYPES OF NUTRIENTS

You may divide food into three groups of nutrients – carbohydrates, fats, and proteins.

Carbohydrates

Carbohydrates are the main source of energy for the body. Your body breaks up carbohydrates into glucose which is then absorbed into the circulation. Blood glucose starts rising within 15 minutes of eating carbohydrates. Carbohydrates are made of starch, sugar, and fiber. Remember that carbohydrates aren't bad. Selecting healthy carbohydrates in appropriate amounts will provide your body with valuable nutrients.

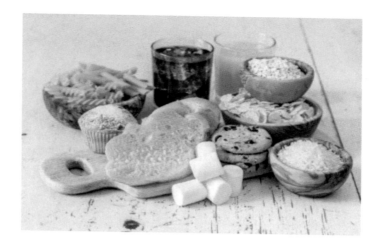

Starch

Foods that are high in starch include vegetables, such as potatoes, peas, corn, lima beans, lentils, pinto beans, and kidney beans, and grains like oat, barley, rice, wheat, pasta, bread, and crackers. The most nutritional kind of grain is whole grain. Whole grains have higher amounts of vitamins, minerals, and fibers than refined grain like rice and white bread. Starchy vegetables and dried beans are also loaded with vitamins and minerals.

Sugars

Examples of natural sugars are fruit and milk while added sugars are those that are used to make cookies, crackers, ice creams, pastries, and pies. Added sugars contain carbohydrates but have little or no nutritional value.

Fiber

Fiber is part of plant foods like vegetables, fruits, nuts, and whole grains. It is a carbohydrate that is not digested and absorbed in the same way as other sugars and starches and has much less effect in raising glucose levels. A high-fiber meal will not raise the glucose in the same way as a low-fiber meal even if both have the same amount of total carbohydrates. Fiber helps you feel full after eating. The American Diabetes Association recommends adults should eat 25-30 grams of fiber per day. It is best to get fiber from food such as fruits and vegetables instead of supplements, as high-fiber foods are also rich in minerals and vitamins.

Sugar Alcohols

Sugar alcohols include reduced calorie sweeteners like mannitol, sorbitol, and xylitol. These are used in sugar free candies and desserts. They do not contain alcohol. They are not always low in carbohydrates and calories. They do not have any advantage in lowering overall glucose control. Excess consumption of sugar alcohols may have a laxative effect leading to gas and diarrhea.

Compare the two nutrition labels. Note that the total carbohydrate is the same on both labels; however, the amount of sugar in the second table is much less than the first one.

NUTRITION FACTS Ice cream bar	
Serving size: 1 Bar (80g)	
Amount per serving	
Total Calories	200
Fat Cal	10
% Daily value	
Total Carbohydrates	21g
Dietary Fiber	0 g
Sugars	18 g

NUTRITION FACTS Ice cream bar	
Serving size: 1 Bar (80g)	
Amount per serving	
Total Calories	200
Fat Cal	10
% Daily value	
Total Carbohydrates	20g
Dietary Fiber	0 g
Sugars	8 g
Sugar alcohol	6g

Artificial Sweeteners

These are non-nutritious sweeteners that may be acceptable substitutes for calorie-containing sweeteners. Non nutritional sweeteners do not appear to have a significant effect on blood glucose.

There are some reports about artificial sweeteners causing cancer but, to date, no study has shown any association between artificial sweeteners and cancer in humans. Six FDA-approved artificial sweeteners are currently used.

SWEETENER	BRAND NAMES
Aspartame	Equal and NutraSweet
Neotame	Neotame
Saccharin	Sweet N' Low and Sugar Twin
Stevia	Purevia, Truvia, and Sun Crystals
Acesulfame	Sunett Sweetener
Sucralose	Splenda

PROTEIN

Proteins are essential nutrients that help our bodies build muscles and tissues. Normally, the body will not use protein for energy unless you do not have enough carbohydrates or fat. Meat, fish, shellfish, egg, and milk, are rich animal sources of proteins. Vegetables, legumes, and grains also have proteins. Nuts like almonds and pistachios and seeds like pine nuts, sunflower, and pumpkin are also rich in proteins.

SOURCES OF PROTEINS

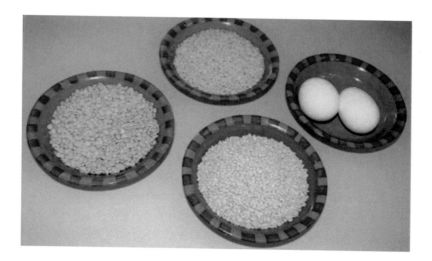

FATS

Fats are essential for the life and functioning of your cells. In addition to fat that you eat, the body makes its own fat called cholesterol. Cholesterol is used to build membranes that protect your cells. Cholesterol is also used for synthesis of various hormones in your body. You only need a small amount of fat in your diet. Fats can be broadly divided in two types: unsaturated fats (Monounsaturated fats & Polyunsaturated fats) and saturated fats.

Unsaturated Fats

Unsaturated fats are liquid at room temperature. These are considered beneficial fats because they improve cholesterol levels, ease inflammation, and stabilize heart rhythm. They are obtained mainly from plant sources such as vegetable oils, nuts, and seeds.

Monounsaturated fats:
Monounsaturated fats are found in olives; oils such as canola and peanut oil; avocados; nuts like almonds, hazel nuts, and pecans; and seeds like pumpkin and sesame.

Polyunsaturated fats:
Polyunsaturated fats are found in vegetable oil such as sunflower, corn oil, soy, cotton seed and nuts like walnuts and flax seed.

Omega-3 fats:
The body cannot make them, so they have to come from food. They're found in fish, walnuts, flax seed, flaxseed oil, and canola or soybean oil.

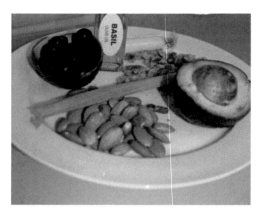

Most people do not eat enough unsaturated fats in their diet. The American Heart Association recommends 8-10 percent of total calories should come from polyunsaturated fats. Evidence shows that increasing the consumption of polyunsaturated fats to 15 percent lowers the risk of heart disease.

Saturated and Trans Fats

Saturated and trans fats, on the other hand, are harmful fats that raise your cholesterol level and cause clogging of the arteries, leading to heart attacks. Saturated fats are found mainly in meat, butter, whole milk, yogurt, ice cream, lard, chocolate, and cream sauces. Turkey and chicken skin, palm oil, coconut oil, and sour cream are other examples of saturated fats. Coconut oil is widely used these days in many diets; however, coconut oil is full of unhealthy saturated fats. Trans fats, found in meat and dairy, are the unhealthiest fats and are mostly made by turning liquid into solid fat. Added to pastries, cookies, and crackers to prolong shelf life, they're often listed as hydrogenated oil or partially hydrogenated oil on food labels. Some examples of foods with trans fats includes cookies, cakes, pastries, muffins, crackers, chips, stick margarine, and shortenings

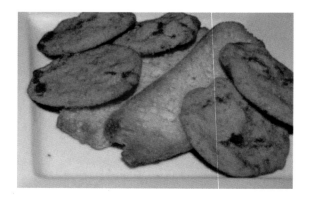

ADOPTING A GOOD NUTRITION PLAN

Now that you have some knowledge about different groups of nutrition, the next step is to formulate a nutrition plan for yourself that suits your lifestyle. To formulate a nutrition plan, it is best to start with a diet diary. Maintaining a diet diary for a few days will give you a good insight into how you are doing with your diet and what changes you need to make. It will also be helpful for you or your dietitian to help formulate a plan. The best meal plan is one that suits your lifestyle as you are more likely to stick to it long term.

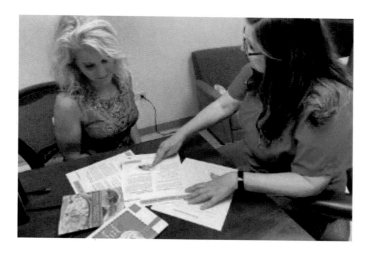

Three ways to formulate a meal plan:

1. The plate method
2. Carb counting
3. Calorie counting

Your goals are specific to you, based on your current weight and your glucose control. Your doctor or dietitian can help you figure out how many carbs per meal you should have and if you need any calorie restriction.

General goals in diabetics are to:

- Keep HbA1c under 7.0
- Keep blood pressure in good control
- Keep total cholesterol and LDL low and increase HDL levels
- Maintain weight to prevent long-term diabetes complications
- Maintain a healthy diet to help you achieve these goals

READING NUTRITION LABELS

Most of the items that you purchase have food labels on them. Food labels are a good source of information on how much carbohydrates, fat, proteins, and calories are present in a food. Two most important things to check are serving size and amount of servings in the container. Remember, information listed on the nutrition label is per serving size so if a container has more than one serving, then you may be consuming much more than what is listed on the label. The second thing to look for is the number of total calories in a serving. The middle portion on a nutrition label will tell you about the nutrients including carbohydrates, proteins, and fats per serving. The amount of nutrients is shown in grams or milligrams and percent daily value.

Nutrition Facts

Serving Size 1 cup (40g)
Serving Per Container 2.5

Amount Per Serving

Calories 150   **Calories from Fat** 10

	% Daily Value*
Total Fat 3g	4%
Saturated Fat 0.5g	2%
Trans Fat 0g	0%
Cholesterol 0mg	0%
Sodium 10mg	1%
Total Carbohydrate 24g	9%
Dietary Fiber 4g	15%
Sugars 1g	
Protein 5g	
Vitamin A	4%
Vitamin C	2%
Calcium	20%
Iron	4%

* Percent Daily Values are based on a 2,000 calorie diet. Your daily values may be higher or lower depending on your calorie needs.

Percent Daily Value

Percent daily value tells you how much of a nutrient in a serving contributes to your daily diet. In general, 5% is considered low and 20% is considered high.

Fats

Fats are listed as total fat, saturated fat, and trans-fat. One should try to avoid picking food with saturated and trans fats because they increase the risk of cardiovascular disease.

Cholesterol and Sodium

Choose items with low cholesterol and sodium to keep your cholesterol and blood pressure in good shape. Sodium is the main ingredient in salt. ADA recommends less than 23 mg, which is equal to one teaspoon of salt per day. People with diabetes have to be cautious about their use of salt, as it leads to high blood pressure.

Carbohydrates

For a person with diabetes, this is the most important part. If you are following a low carbohydrate diet, extra attention should be paid to the amount of carbs per serving.

Vitamins and Minerals

Americans do not take enough vitamins and minerals in their diet. The best way to get them is by eating a balanced diet. You do not need supplementation unless you are deficient, and your doctor recommends that you supplement. ADA does not specifically recommend taking fish oil tablets or vitamins. Instead, it recommends having fish and flax seed.

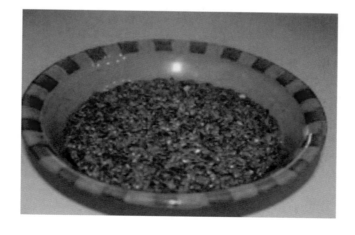

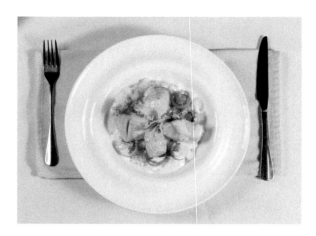

PORTION SIZING

It is important to eat not only the right type of food but also the right amount. Consistent and balanced meals are an important part of blood glucose control. Portion control can be the most difficult thing to do as your brain is programmed to eat until you are completely stuffed instead of stopping when you are not hungry anymore. A portion is the amount of certain food that you choose to eat. On the positive side, portion control can allow you to eat a wide variety of food that you love.

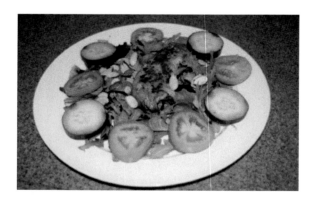

Plate Method

The balanced plate is an easy and effective way to do portion sizing in the plate method. You divide your plate into four portions and fill each portion with a different group of food. Ideally, two portions of the plate should be non-starchy vegetables and one of the remaining small portions would be starch, like whole grains and other small portions would be protein such as chicken, turkey, or fish. If you are planning to drink juice, yogurt, or milk along with your meal, this will add to the carbohydrate portion.

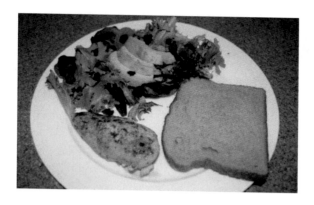

CARBOHYDRATE COUNTING

Carb counting is the recommended and most popular way for diabetics to plan their diet. Low carb diets have gained much popularity in people with or without diabetes. It is important to understand that carb counting is not the same as a low carb diet. With carb counting, you keep track of the amount of carbohydrates you eat with each meal. If you are doing carb counting, that does not mean you go overboard with the amount of protein and fat, as that will add more calories. Too many calories will offset the benefits of doing carb counting. Doing carb counting does not mean completely eliminating carbohydrates from the diet as carbs are an important source of energy for the body.

Counting and eating a planned amount of carbohydrates will help manage your glucose levels in goal range. Variations in amounts of carbs taken throughout the day, such as eating a big meal or skipping a meal, will lead to wide fluctuations in blood glucose. It is important to eat a balanced amount of carbs with each meal.

The American Diabetes Association does not recommend a specific amount of carbohydrates to be taken with each meal. In general, the recommendation is to have 45 carbs per meal for women and 60 carbs per meal for men. This will vary, depending on the weight of the person and glucose levels. The biggest advantage of carb counting is that it allows you to enjoy a variety of carbs as long as you are eating within the allowance suggested. One may think carb counting might be a lot of work. However, it is not as hard as it sounds.

In today's world, almost every pre-packaged meal has the amount of carbs and calories listed on it. When buying ingredients, one can look at the nutritional label for total amount of carbs. It is important to remember that the total carbs listed on the nutrition label is only the amount of carbs in one serving. If you're planning to have more than one serving, you have to multiply the amount of carbs by the number of servings. Sometimes carbs are referred to as serving size. Each carb serving is equal to 15 grams of carbs. If you are eating fresh food, you can easily get the carbohydrate information from various books and online and mobile apps.

Several carb counting apps are available on smartphones. All you have to do is log in the information of what you are eating and the app will calculate the total amount of carbs and calories for you.

For years, people with diabetes were advised to completely give up on sweets. Now, with better understanding of diabetes in the last 2 decades, we know that although different types of food will affect your blood glucose differently, it is the total amount of carbs that matters. If you are planning to have a piece of cake or dessert for your meal, you may want to minimize the other carbs in your plate and replace it with more veggies.

Tips for Cutting Back on Carbs

- Replace white bread with wheat bread
- Eat an open-faced sandwich
- Replace bread with lettuce in your sandwich
- Replace the sugar in your tea, coffee, or baked goods with an artificial sweetener or avoid using added sugar at all

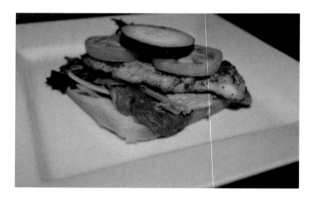

Glycemic Index

Another important concept is glycemic index, which is the ranking of carbohydrate-containing food based on their effects on blood glucose. Food with a high glycemic index will raise blood glucose more than food with low glycemic index, even if the total amount of carbohydrates is the same. Using glycemic index as the guide for meal planning is very difficult, as it is affected by many other factors. Glycemic index is mostly used for research purposes. It is not practical to use in day-to-day diet planning. The American Diabetes Association does not recommend any specific meal plan based on glycemic index meal planning.

ADVANCED CARBOHYDRATE COUNTING

Once you have learned the basics about carb counting, you can move on to learning advanced carb counting. This requires more skill and learning. A dietitian or diabetes educator will be able to help you learn advanced carb counting. This involves learning pattern management for your blood glucose and adjusting your mealtime insulin dose based on the amount of carbs in your meal and your glucose levels.

Calculating Insulin Dose Based on Carb and Correction

This is a two-step process:

1. A calculation from carb intake based on insulin-to-carb ratio
2. Correcting for high glucose based on correction factor

Most people need 1 unit of insulin to cover for 10 grams of carbs; however, this ratio can vary and can be calculated, depending on an individual's weight, activity, and records of food intake. For example, if your insulin-to-carb ratio is 1:10, you take 1 unit of insulin for every 10 grams you eat. Based on this, if you are planning to eat 60 grams of carb, your insulin dose will be 6 units. You then look at your blood glucose levels and correct for high glucose. This is done by calculating insulin sensitivity factor. This is a calculated value and varies in different individuals. Your doctor or diabetes educator can calculate your insulin sensitivity and give you the ratio. To calculate the correction factor, you subtract your goal glucose from the total glucose and divide the result by your insulin sensitivity factor. For example, if your insulin sensitivity is 30, your glucose level is 200, and target glucose 120, then your correction is calculated as 210-120= 90/30 =3

Your total insulin dose = dose from carb counting plus correction is 6+3 =9 units.

MEAL PLANNING

Diet Diary

It has been observed that most people underestimate the amount of food they eat by 20-30%. To give yourself and your dietitian a better idea of what you are eating, maintaining a diet diary where you would log in everything you eat or drink for 3-5 days is recommended. This will give you a good idea of what kind of food you are eating and what needs to be replaced. Include all beverages in your diet diary. Drinking juices, milk, soda, and other flavored beverages can add a lot of extra calories to your meal. Planning a meal ahead of time greatly helps to cut down the calories and helps to make better choices. While planning, keep your goals in mind.

Making a Shopping List

Here are some tips for smart shopping:

- Make a list to shop. It will prevent you from picking unnecessary snacks and food
- Do not shop when you are hungry. When you are hungry, you are much more likely to pick up unhealthy snacks
- When picking packaged foods like bread or pasta, make sure you look at the nutrition label, total carbs, fiber, and serving sizes
- Pick up a lot of green vegetables. You are more likely to use them if you have them around you
- Consider picking nuts for salads and snacking

Once you are done with shopping, the next step is to see how you can prepare your meal in the healthiest way.

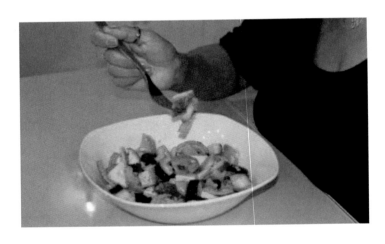

Tips for Healthy Cooking

- Try to chop your vegetables in advance. It is easier to use them for snacks and in cooking if they're ready to eat
- Try baking or steaming your meals instead of frying
- Use olive oil or canola oil instead of corn or coconut oil
- Try to make homemade salad dressings.
- Add lemon or lemon zest ginger and herbs to flavor your food
- Change your recipes by subtracting unhealthy ingredients and replacing with more healthy ones
- Add one or two serving of vegetables to your pasta and other recipes

MEALTIME HABITS

Review your meal time habits. How many meals and snacks are you having and how frequently? It is important that diabetics who take medication do not skip meals and that the meals are spaced at appropriate intervals. Not every diabetic needs two to three snacks. If you are a snacker, make more healthy choices like vegetables or fruits. It is advisable that you have a meal at the kitchen table and avoid doing other activities like watching TV or browsing through your phone while eating, as it will distract you and lead you to eat more calories. Here are some choices for healthy snacking.

Healthy Snacks Less than 5 Grams of Carbs:

- 10 almonds
- 15 peanuts
- 5 baby carrots
- 1 cup light popcorn
- 1 string of string cheese
- 10 goldfish crackers

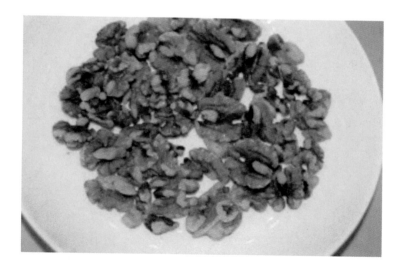

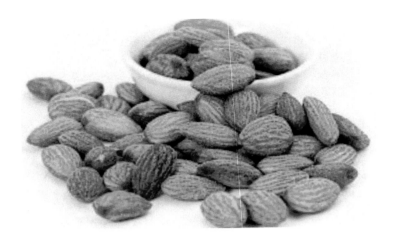

Healthy Snacks 10-15 Grams of Carbs

- One small apple
- One small orange
- ½ cup hummus
- 1 cup fresh veggies
- ¼ cup dried fruit
- ¼ cup cottage cheese

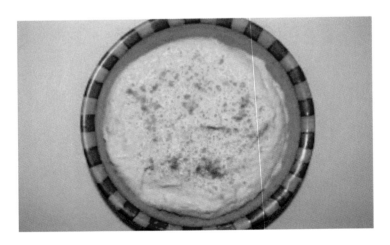

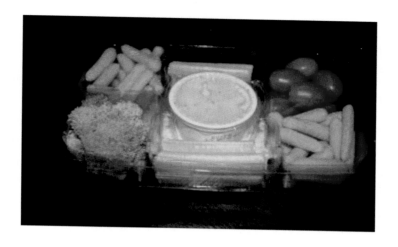

EATING OUT

The idea of eating out is fun, but it can be very challenging for a person with diabetes as you do not have much control over the ingredients used. Today, most restaurants offer a low carb and healthy heart menu. Additionally, many dishes on the menu have nutritional information listed. Most restaurants allow you to replace ingredients or sides on your dish, like replacing rice or pasta with vegetables

Fast food places also have many healthy choices, and nutritional information is available on the drive-thru menus and online.

Tips for Healthy Fast Food

- Replace bread with lettuce
- Eat sandwiches with wheat bread or low-carb wraps
- Order junior sizes
- Avoid supersizing
- Choose roasted or grilled options instead of fried
- Skip cheese. If counting calories, this will save 100 calories per meal
- Add vegetables
- Choose white meat or fish over red meat
- Choose brown rice over white rice or noodles
- Consider sharing your entrée

If you're a diabetic on a diabetic medication, especially mealtime insulin, it's important to take it on time to avoid a spike in your glucose levels. If your meal is going to be delayed, you may want to take a small snack to avoid hypoglycemia.

DRINKS AND ALCOHOLIC BEVERAGES

People with diabetes wonder if alcohol is okay. It is best to discuss with your doctor if you can have a drink or two, as certain diabetes medication may interact with alcohol. Also, if you have elevated triglyceride levels along with high glucose levels, it may be advisable to avoid drinking alcohol as that will greatly exacerbate your blood glucose levels. Soft drinks and alcoholic beverages are often not taken into consideration when counting calories. Drinks can be a significant source of sugar and calories, contributing to an increase in blood glucose and weight.

The American Diabetes Association recommends sugar free, calorie free drinks like water, unsweetened tea, or coffee. If you like some flavor, you can add fresh lemon or lime, raspberries, strawberries, or orange to your water.

For most diabetics, it is okay to drink alcohol in moderation, which translates to having one drink per day for all women and for men over age 65 and two drinks per day for men under age 65. One drink equals one 12 ounce can of beer, which is 150 calories, one 5-ounce glass of wine, which is 100 calories, or a 1.5-ounce shot of liquor. It is recommended to always drink with food. Never drink on an empty stomach due to risk of hypoglycemia. Alcohol can lower blood glucose up to 12 hours. Make sure you check your blood glucose level before going to bed if you have had an alcoholic beverage. Although one should never drink and drive, drinking combined with the risk of hypoglycemia can be very dangerous for everyone on the road. Alcohol also has calories. Make sure you add this to your calorie count. To cut back on calories from alcohol, use low or no calorie mixers such as diet soda, a club soda, or water. Put less liquor in your drink and choose light beer over regular beer.

Water, by all means, is the best drink. It is refreshing, cheap, and calorie free. It keeps you well hydrated and improves brain function and energy. Water has also been shown to reduce headaches. Drinking water prevents conditions like constipation and kidney stones and helps prevent hangovers. There is also some evidence that increasing water intake can promote weight loss by increasing metabolism.

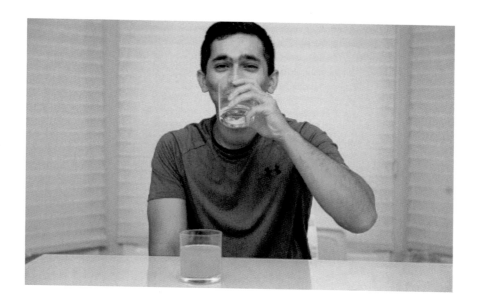

Chapter 5

PHYSICAL ACTIVITY

Physical activity is like a secret weapon to help fight diabetes. Exercise is one of the best things you can do for your mind and body. Exercise can directly affect your diabetes by lowering your blood glucose levels. When you exercise, your body becomes more sensitive to insulin. This can significantly lower the amount of medication or insulin you need to take control of your blood glucose. The terms "exercise" and "physical activity" are often used interchangeably. There is a difference between physical activity and exercise. The former means any activity that results in energy expenditure; however, exercise refers to a more vigorous activity involving increase in heart rate, breathing, and perspiration.

BENEFITS OF EXERCISE IN DIABETES

- Lowers blood glucose levels and increases insulin sensitivity
- Reduces the need for insulin and other diabetic medications
- Lowers your cholesterol levels
- Lowers blood pressure
- Strengthens your heart muscle and lowers your risk of heart disease and stroke
- Promotes weight loss and prevents weight gain
- Strengthens your bones, improves strength, flexibility, and endurance
- Improves brain function and mood
- Helps fight stress
- Increases your energy levels for daily activity
- Helps you sleep better. People who exercise have better quality and quantity of sleep
- Improves balance and prevents falls
- Reduces symptoms of depression and improves quality of life. Exercise releases certain chemicals called endorphins, which makes you feel good and boosts your mood

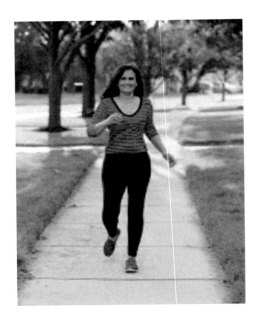

The American Diabetes Association recommends people with diabetes have at least 30 minutes of moderate intensity exercise 5 days a week. It is also recommended that people with diabetes should sit less. Staying physically active does not necessarily mean going to the gym and working out on a machine. There are several different ways one can be physically active. Every small movement counts. When you are sitting more, you must get up every 30 minutes for 3-4 minutes and move around. This will improve not only your glucose level but also your circulation and prevent complications like having a blood clot in your legs.

Examples of Physical Activity That One Can do Without Going to the Gym

- Taking stairs instead of elevators
- Parking your car far away in parking lots
- Walking a dog
- Lawn mowing
- Working in the yard
- Standing frequently then sitting, for example, when talking on the phone, standing up and moving around instead of sitting in one place
- Taking your kids to the park
- Sweeping the floors or the patio
- Incorporating walking in your daily activities
- Moving around during commercial breaks while watching TV

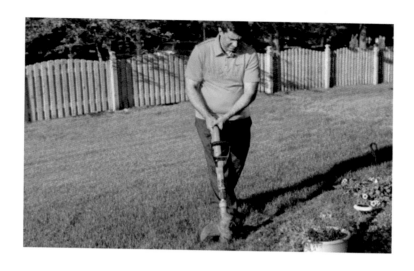

SETTING UP A MINDSET

Like anything else, setting up a mindset and preparing yourself first for staying physically active will encourage you to stick to your plan. Have a conversation with yourself about how staying active will help you stay healthy in the long run. Visualize yourself being able to do activities and playing around with your kids and grandkids like you would like you to do. Visualize being able to travel the world and do things you enjoy. This will motivate you to keep going.

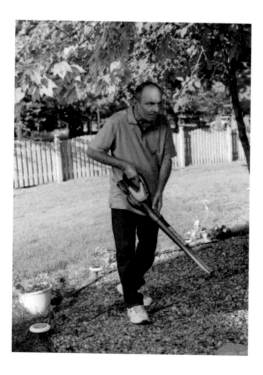

GETTING STARTED

Talk to your healthcare provider before you start any exercise program or any fitness or exercise regimen, depending upon the type of activity you are planning to do. Your provider may order some tests such as a stress test to check your heart and blood vessels before you start an exercise program, especially if you already have complications from diabetes. If you are currently not exercising, start exercise slowly and gradually increase your activity level as tolerated. For example, if you have not been walking and are now planning to walk regularly, start with 10 to 15 minutes of walking per day for a few days and then add 5 to 10 minutes every day. Same with exercising. Start slowly and increase activity as tolerated, as doing too much too fast can lead to injuries and could keep you away from exercising altogether, and it will also discourage you to continue exercising if you are feeling uncomfortable.

TYPES OF PHYSICAL ACTIVITY

Choosing the right type of exercises is important. For some, walking every day is the best thing they can do, but others can get involved in more moderate to severe strenuous activity.

Personal fitness score. Your choice of activity will also depend on what you are trying to achieve. Most people with diabetes share a personal goal of lowering HbA1c and losing weight. Your goal does not have to be related to diabetes. You may have a goal of looking a certain way. You may have a goal of losing weight or building muscle mass.

Walking

Walking is one of the easiest and inexpensive physical activities to do. It's safe and simple and has many health benefits.

Benefits of Walking

- It could help reduce your risk of diabetes
- It helps control your glucose if you already have diabetes
- It reduces the risk of heart attack
- It reduces the risk of high blood pressure and stroke
- It manages stress and depression
- It helps improve circulation and maintains bone density

Walking Shoes

Wearing proper walking shoes is also very important, especially for diabetics. It is imperative to make sure your shoes are comfortable and fit properly to avoid any injuries to your feet. Diabetics tend to have calluses and corns on their feet, which might get rubbed with poorly fitted shoes and become a source of infection. In the United States, diabetics who are on Medicare are eligible to get one pair of customized walking shoes per year after getting a recommendation from their health care provider and podiatrist. Some private insurance companies will also cover diabetic shoes.

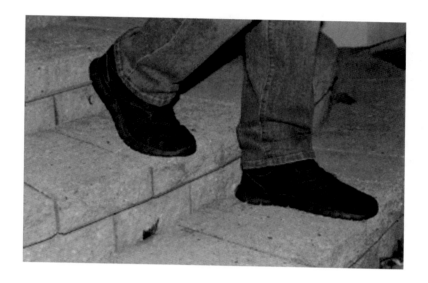

EXERCISE

Aerobic Exercise

You may have heard the terms 'aerobic' and 'anaerobic' when it comes to exercise.

Aerobic exercises are activities includes those activities that use oxygen, increasing your heart rate and getting your large muscles moving.

Some examples of aerobic activity include:
- Walking
- Cardio
- Swimming
- Jogging
- Skiing
- Dancing
- Playing tennis
- Biking

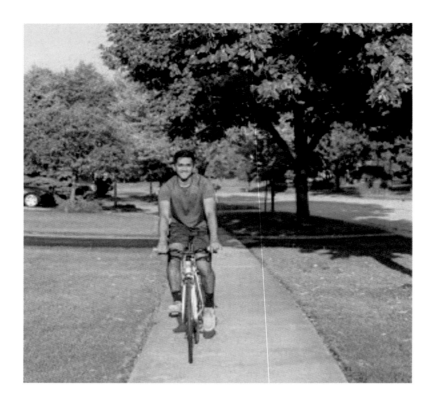

Aerobic activity is awesome for diabetes, as it increases your muscles to take glucose from the blood and thereby lowering blood glucose levels. It also increases the utilization of glucose for energy, making cells more sensitive to insulin. Aerobic activity also helps burn calories and maintain weight.

Anaerobic Exercise

Anaerobic exercise lowers glucose without using oxygen. Anaerobic activity involves quick bursts of intense activity for a shorter length of time. For example, jumping or heavy weight lifting. During anaerobic activity, your body uses stored energy instead of oxygen. Anaerobic activity is good for building muscle and losing weight. Anaerobic activity can also improve bone strength and decrease the feeling of depression. The main difference between aerobic and anaerobic exercise is the intensity at which one is working out.

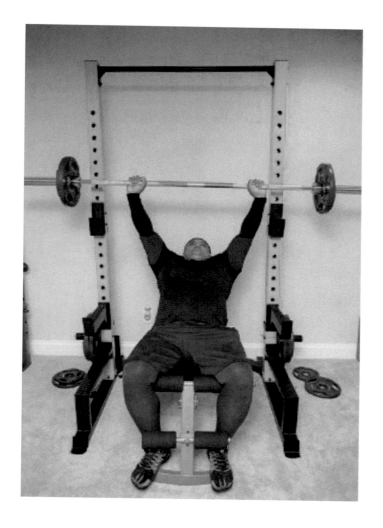

Strength Training

Includes the use of free weights and resistance bands. You have to be careful when starting weight training as incorrect use of weights or improper posture during resistance training can lead to serious injuries.

Benefits of Resistance Training

Benefits of resistance training include improvement in muscle mass, body composition, muscle strength, bone mineral density, insulin sensitivity, blood pressure, lipids, and cardiovascular health. Start training with lifting small amounts of weight, one to two pounds and gradually increase as your endurance builds up. It is important to breathe while lifting weights as blood pressure may rise to dangerous levels if you do not breathe. Give your body time to recover between workouts. Focus on a different muscle group each time.

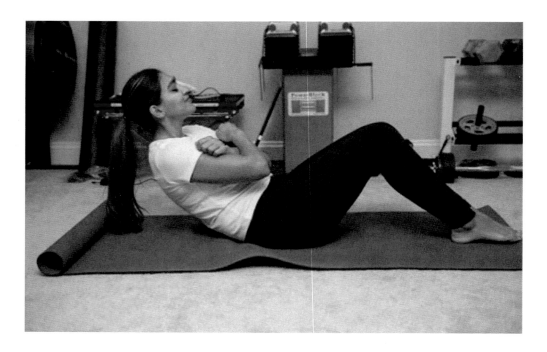

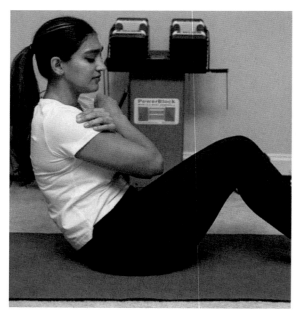

Stretching and Balance Exercises

Stretching and balance exercises are activities that stretch your muscles and joints and help maintain positive posture and balance. These include activities like yoga and pilates. Stretching exercises can be easily done at home, as it requires minimal or no equipment. Stretching exercises are good for older people as they can increase the range of motion, joint flexibility, and balance.

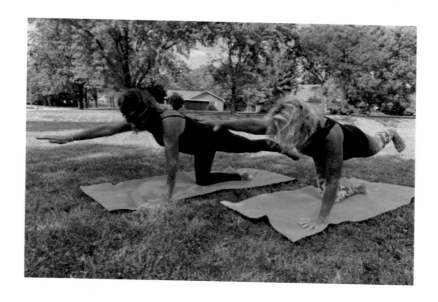

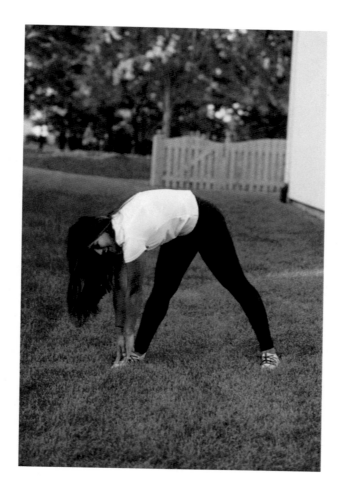

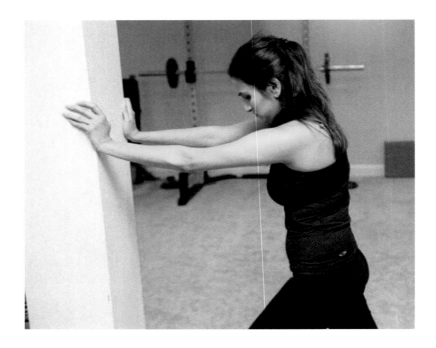

Warming Up and Cooling Down

Warming up before you start any exercise is extremely important. Prepare your body first. Regardless of what kind of exercise you do, start with a slow pace and gradually increase your intensity. For example, if you are jogging, start with basic walking. If you are running, start with jogging. If on a treadmill, start with a slower speed for the first few minutes. The same pattern of gradually warming up applies to finishing exercise or cooling down.

PERSONALIZED WORKOUT PLAN

Each person's goal for working out should be based on their age, current health status, and comorbidities. You can go to a gym and have a personalized trainer. That certainly helps. However, you can easily have a personalized exercise plan based on the activities that you can do on your own.

Getting started with an exercise regimen is often the most important and most difficult step. Once you start, you just have to continue motivating yourself to keep going. Pick one to two activities from each type of exercise. For example, after warming up, walk or jog for 15 to 20 minutes, followed by stress training for 10 to 15 minutes, followed by stretching with cooling down. Alternatively, you can also pick each type of activity 2 days a week. Whatever activity you choose must be the one you enjoy doing.

How do you keep motivated? Even people who are committed to exercise will lose motivation once in a while. To stay motivated, make an exercise plan for yourself and write it down, especially if you are not going to a gym. Have a realistic goal. Have a clear idea of how many days in a week you want to work out and for how long. Also, try to set up a time for your workout so you can plan your other activities around it. Track your progress, find a partner to work out with you.

Exercise can lower blood glucose levels, but it can also put some people at a higher risk of hyperglycemia. It is recommended that you check your blood glucose level before starting any exercise and after you are done working out. If your glucose is low (for most people, below 100) before you start, then you may want to take a small snack. If you are exercising for a longer time, sometimes, you may have to check your glucose in between activities. A glucose level of 100 to 250 is safe for most people to exercise. If your glucose is over 300 it is generally recommended not to exercise before you bring your glucose down because of the risk of increasing the glucose even more.

WHEN IS THE BEST TIME TO EXERCISE FOR DIABETICS?

The best time to exercise will vary on an individual basis, depending upon what diabetes medications you are on. If you are on insulin, you may not want to exercise up to 2-3 hours after injecting fast acting insulin due to risk of hypoglycemia. You may need adjustment in your insulin dose if you are planning to exercise after a meal. For those who are on oral medications, exercising after meals might be safe when your blood glucose level is high.

Chapter 6

PHARMACOLOGICAL MANAGEMENT OF DIABETES

Lifestyle modification with diet and exercise is the key to management of diabetes. Several studies have proven that lifestyle modification can lower the risk of diabetes and development of complications by 50%. Lifestyle modification is usually enough for prediabetes, but once you develop diabetes, most people will be needing some diabetes medication to keep the blood glucose in normal range. Maintaining your blood glucose in the normal range is very important, as it will prevent long-term complications. The good news is that diabetes research has made tremendous progress in the last 10 to 15 years. Today, we know more about diabetes than ever before.

In this chapter, we'll review all the diabetes medications currently available and FDA approved in the United States. We'll discuss how each medicine works and its benefits and possible side effects. Most people who are diagnosed with Type 2 diabetes are started on oral medications first. However, the choice of medication really depends on your blood glucose level at the time of diagnosis, how long you have been diabetic, what your current glucose level is, and what complications you already have. Diabetes treatment is customized for every individual and, therefore, no two people can be compared with each other. For example, a medication that is working for a friend or family member may not be a good choice for you. And vice versa. Similarly, if you know someone has developed a certain side effect from a diabetes medication, it does not mean that you will also develop the same side effect.

Your health care provider is the best person to discuss your medications. You must never discontinue any medication on your own, thinking it is not working or because of the side effects, without discussing with a healthcare provider. It is important to have some knowledge about the medication you are using regarding how it works, what possible side effects it could have, and what kind of monitoring it requires. Do not hesitate to ask these questions to your doctor when started on any new medication. Also, know the names of your medication. Always carry your medication list with you and update your list with current doses when you see your doctor.

TYPES OF DIABETES MEDICATIONS

There are several different classes of diabetes medication available today.

- Oral medications in pill forms
- Non-insulin injectable medications
- Insulins that are mostly injectable
- Inhaled insulin

ORAL DIABETES MEDICATIONS

Several different classes of diabetes medications are available. Medications are divided into different classes based on how they work. Each class may have several different brands of medication made by different companies. We'll use both brand names and generic names to avoid any confusion. Brand names are based on the company that is making the medication.

Nine different classes of oral medications are currently available for management of Type 2 diabetes in the United States. These classes are as follows:

Classes of Oral Diabetes Medication

- Biguanide
- Sulfonylurea
- DPP-4 Inhibitors
- SGLT-2 Inhibitors
- Meglitinides
- Thiozolididiones
- Alpha Glucosidase Inhibitors
- Bile acid sequestrants
- Dopamine agonist

BIGUANIDES

Drugs included in this class

- Metformin (Glucophage)
- Glucophage XR
- Fortamet
- Riomet (liquid formulation)

Metformin

Metformin is the most commonly prescribed diabetes medication all over the world. The American Diabetes Association and American Association of Clinical Endocrinologists both recommend metformin as the first line agent for treatment of diabetes. It can also be used in the treatment of prediabetes. Metformin was first approved by the FDA in 1990. The brand name for metformin is Glucophage. It is available in tablet form and in liquid form and can be taken once or twice a day depending on the dose prescribed by your doctor. Glucophage XR is an extended release version of metformin.

How Does Metformin Work?

Metformin works by making your body more sensitive to your own insulin, so more glucose is used as energy. It also helps your liver release glucose more slowly. Unlike some other medications, it does not make your body release more insulin and, therefore, does not cause episodes of low sugar. Other forms of metformin include Fortamet and Riomet, which is the liquid form of metformin.

Metformin is one of the strongest pills available for diabetes. Studies have shown metformin lowers HbA1c by 1.5%. In addition, it is not associated with weight gain and has been shown to help with weight loss by decreasing the insulin resistance.

Possible Side Effects

Some of the common side effects associated with metformin are diarrhea and nausea. These side effects are dose dependent and in most people subside in a few weeks. In some cases, diarrhea may persist and you may need a lower dose or you may be unable to take it. Side effects are more common with higher doses of medication. Other side effects are bloating, gas, headache, metallic taste in the mouth, lactic acidosis, and vitamin B 12 deficiency. Lactic acidosis is a rare side effect which causes muscle pain. It can occur in patients with kidney disease and with use of alcohol. Patients using metformin should be cautious with drinking alcohol as it can precipitate lactic acidosis. Long term use of metformin can cause vitamin B12 deficiency. Levels should be monitored periodically in patients using metformin.

Renal Function Monitoring

Metformin should be used cautiously in patients with chronic kidney disease. Based on current recommendations, metformin should not be used if the GFR is less than 40 and creatinine is more than 1.50. Metformin should also not be used in patients with class 4 heart failure.

Much confusion exists regarding metformin and kidney disease. Sometimes people are scared to even start metformin due to fear of damaging the kidneys. It is very important to understand that metformin does not cause kidney damage. But if your kidneys are not functioning properly and you already have some degree of kidney damage due to diabetes, high BP, or some other reason, then using metformin might make it worse. Your doctor should be monitoring your kidney function periodically. It is generally recommended to stop metformin for one day prior to undergoing any procedures that involves use of IV dye like angiograms or CT scans.

SULFONYLUREAS

This is one of the oldest classes of diabetes medication. It was first approved in 1950. It was the second most widely used medication for diabetes until a few years ago. In the past decade, with the availability of several other new classes of medications, the use of sulfonylureas has significantly declined.

Following are the drugs in Sulfonylurea class.

- Amaryl (Glimeperide)
- Glucotrol (Glipizide)
- Diabeta (Glyburide)
- Glynase (Glyburide)
- Glycron (Glyburide)
- Diabinese (Chlorpropamide)
- Tol-tab (Tolbutamide)

How Does Sulfonylurea Work?

Sulfonylurea works by stimulating your pancreas to make more insulin, which, in turn, lowers your glucose levels. For sulfonylureas to work, your pancreas must be capable of making insulin.

Possible Side Effects

Since sulfonylureas work by increasing the release of insulin, they're notorious for causing low blood glucose, especially if you have impaired liver or kidney function. If you are having frequent low glucose reactions, then your sulfonylurea dose may have to be adjusted, or you may have to switch to a different medication.

Other side effects of sulfonylureas include weight gain, rashes, and upset stomach. Risk of hypoglycemia with sulfonylurea is also increased when used with alcohol and other drugs like decongestants. On the other hand, medications like steroids can decrease the effect of sulfonylureas. Because so many new medications are now available that do not cause severe hypoglycemia and have additional benefits, sulfonylureas are not prescribed as much as before.

MEGLITINIDES

Drugs included in this class:

- Repaglinide (Prandin)
- Nateglinide (Starlix)

How Does Meglitinide Work?

Meglitinides works similarly as sulfonylurea by stimulating the pancreas to make more insulin. However, it works much faster and is eliminated from the body in 3-4 hours. Because of the shorter duration of action, they're usually taken three times a day before meals.

Possible Side Effects

Most common side effect is low blood glucose, upset stomach, headache, and weight gain.

DPP-4 INHIBITORS

Drugs included in this class

- Sitagliptin (Januvia)
- Saxagliptin (Onglyza)
- Alogliptin (Nesina)
- Linagliptin (Tradgenta)

How do DPP-4 Inhibitors Work?

DPP-4 inhibitors belong to the incretin group of hormones. Incretins are hormones that signal the body to release insulin after eating.

GLP-1 is one such hormone, but the body breaks down this hormone quickly after it is released. DPP-4 inhibitors inhibit the enzyme which breaks down GLP-1, thereby allowing GLP-1 to linger around, dropping glucose levels. These are relatively mild medications and lower HbA1c by 0.5% maximum. These drugs are used in treatment of mild diabetes or in combination with other diabetic medications.

Possible Side Effects

Upper respiratory tract infections, joint pains, headache, sore throat, inflammation of the pancreas, and GI symptoms like nausea, vomiting, or diarrhea.

SGLT-2 INHIBITORS
(sodium glucose co-transporter-2 inhibitors)

Drugs included in this class

- Empagliflozin (Jardiance)
- Canagliflozin (Invokana)
- Dapagliflozin (Farxiga)
- Ertugliflozin (Steglatro)

How do SGLT-2 Inhibitors Work?

This is a unique class of medication that works very differently from most other oral medications. The first SGLT-2 inhibitor was approved in 2013. SGLT-2 inhibitors work by helping the kidneys to dump excess glucose in urine. They block the receptors in the kidneys that would normally allow glucose to be absorbed.

Other Benefits of SGLT-2 Inhibitors

- They promote significant weight loss
- Help reduce blood pressure
- Decrease the risk of cardiovascular disease
- Decrease the rate of hospitalization in heart-failure patients

Most of the medications in this class have proven cardiovascular benefits in clinical trials. Because of this additional benefit, the use of SGLT-2 inhibitors have been significantly increasing.

Possible Side Effects

One of the biggest drawbacks of SGLT-2 inhibitors is that because it works through the kidneys, the renal function has to be above a certain level for a person to be able to use these medications. Because they work by spilling more glucose into the urine, they're more prone to cause genital yeast infection and urinary tract infection. These drugs are generally not advised for patients who have a history of recurrent urinary tract infections or genital yeast infections. They may also cause diabetic ketoacidosis. People with bladder cancer should not use Farxiga. They are also available in combination pills with DPP-4 inhibitors and Metformin.

THIAZOLIDINEDIONES

Drugs included in this class

- Rosiglitazone (Avandia)
- Pioglitazone (Actos)

How Does Thiazolidinediones Work?

Thiazolidinediones medication increases insulin sensitivity and helps with increasing the utilization of glucose in the body, thereby lowering blood glucose levels. Thiazolidinediones were first approved in 1990. They also have additional benefits with lipid lowering. They were very popular medications until 2010 when Avandia was shown to be associated with increased risk of heart attack. However, in 2013, FDA removed these restrictions. Rosiglitazone is also shown to be associated with increased risk of fractures. Pioglitazone is associated with bladder cancer and it is contraindicated in patients with bladder issues. Other side effects include increased fluid retention and weight gain. Because of the side effect profile, the use of these medications has considerably declined in the last decade.

GLP-1 AGONIST

Drug included in this class

- Rybelsus (Semaglutide)

Rybelsus is the only oral GLP-1 agent approved recently. All the other GLP-1 agents are administered via subcutaneous injection. Rybelsus comes in a 3-mg dose which is to be continued for four weeks; the dose is then increased to 7 mg and can be titrated up to 14 mg if needed. Detailed mechanism of action and side effect profile of GLP-1 class of medication will be discussed later in this chapter.

ALPHA GLUCOSIDASE INHIBITOR

Drugs included in this class

- Acarbose (precose)
- Miglitol (glyset)

These medications work differently than other medications. They're not used frequently.

How do Alpha Glucosidase Inhibitors Work?

Alpha glucosidase inhibitors work by slowing down the absorption of glucose from the intestine after you eat. They're taken before a meal. They lower the sharp rise in glucose after a meal.

Possible Side Effects

Include bloating, gas, and diarrhea.

BILE ACID SEQUESTRANTS

Drugs included in this class

- Colveselam (welchol)

How do Bile Sequestrants Work?

These are cholesterol lowering medications that were also found to lower blood glucose. Mechanism of action how bile acid sequestrants lower glucose is not clearly understood.

Possible Side Effects

Includes upset stomach, constipation, nausea.

DOPAMINE AGONIST

Drugs included in this class

- Cycloset (Bromocriptine mesylate)

How do Dopamine Agonists Work?

These are medications that work by boosting the release of a chemical called dopamine in the brain. It is not clear how this helps to reduce blood glucose levels.

Cycloset is an FDA approved for diabetes and works primarily in the brain. It has to be taken within 2 hours of waking up.

Possible Side Effects

Low blood pressure, fainting, dizziness, and upset stomach

COMBINATION PILLS

Several of the oral pills discussed above are also available in combination with each other.

List of Combination pills

- Metformin and Glipizide   (Metaglip)
- Metformin and Glyburide   (Glucovance)
- Metformin and Sitagliptin   (Janumet)
- Metformin and Linagliptin   (Jentadeuto)
- Metformin and Prandin   (PrandiMet)
- Metformin and Dapagliflozin   (Xigduo)
- Metformin and Empagliflozin   (Synjardy)
- Metformin and Invokana   (Invokamet)
- Metformin and Pioglitazone   (Actosplusmet)
- Metformin and Rosiglitazone   (Avandamet).
- Metformin and Alogliptin   (Kazano)
- Dapagliflozin and Saxagliptin   (Qtern)
- Empagliflozin and Linagliptin   (Glyxambi)
- Alogliptin and Pioglitazone   (Oseni)
- Metformin and Saxagliptin   (Kombiglyze)

INJECTABLE MEDICATIONS

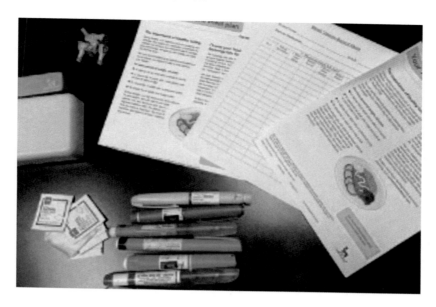

GLP-1 AGONIST (Glucagon like peptide-1)

How do GLP Analogs Work?

Glucagon-like peptide analogs are also called incretin mimetics because they mimic the action of incretin hormones in your body and help lower your glucose levels. GLP agonist can be used with oral diabetes pills as well as with insulin. Research has shown that these medications have other health benefits in addition to lowering glucose such as lowering blood pressure, weight reduction, decreasing cholesterol levels, and beta cell preservation.

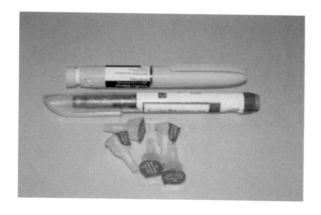

GLP Agonists Work in Different Parts of the Body.

- They lower blood glucose by mimicking the action of incretin hormones
- In the brain, GLP-1 sends signals to the hypothalamus to take less water and food, increasing satiety, which leads to weight loss
- In the muscle, GLP-1 stimulates new glucose formation and increases glucose uptake by the cells
- In the pancreas, GLP-1 stimulates the pancreas to release more insulin, decreasing the amount of post-meal glycogen
- In the pancreas, it also decreases the amount of glucagon, which is a hormone that increases glucose levels in the liver
- In the liver, GLP-1 decreases hepatic glucose output, thus lowering the amount of glucose in the blood
- In the stomach, GLP-1 slows down the passage of food, prolonging the sensation of fullness resulting in early satiety and weight loss. It also decreases the secretion of acid in the stomach

TYPES OF GLP-1 RECEPTOR AGONIST

There are two different types of GLP-1 receptor agonist: short acting GLP-1, which has to be taken once or twice daily, and long-acting GLP-1, which is taken once a week.

List of Currently Available GLP-1 Agents

Short acting

- Victoza taken once daily
- Byetta taken twice a day

Long-Acting

- Bydureon taken once a week
- Ozempic taken once a week
- Trulicity taken once a week

GLP-1 also comes in combination with insulin.

GLP-1/ Insulin Combinations

- Soliqua (Insulin Glargine/Lixisenatide)
- Xultophy (Insulin Degludec/Liraglutide)

Byetta

Exenetide was the first GLP drug approved in 2005. It was discovered from the saliva of a Gila monster lizard. The short acting version of exenatide is Byetta, which is administered by subcutaneous injection twice a day. Byetta promotes insulin production after a meal but only if glucose is high. Since it does not work when glucose is low, it does not cause hypoglycemia. Byetta comes in prefilled pens in two different doses, 5 mg and 10 mg.

Possible Side Effects

The most common side effect with Byetta is nausea, which improves with time. Other possible side effects include vomiting, diarrhea, headache, and risk for pancreatitis.

Liraglutide (Victoza)

Liraglutide like exenatide also works by mimicking the action of GLP-1 hormone.

It stimulates insulin production when blood glucose levels are high.

- Decreases glucagon production
- Delays stomach emptying
- Liraglutide also comes in a prefilled pen and is injected once a day

Possible Side Effects

Include nausea, diarrhea, and increased risk of pancreatitis.

Pramlintide (Symlin)

Pramlintide works by mimicking the action of hormone Amlin, which is secreted by the pancreas and increases the release of insulin by the beta cells in the pancreas.

Possible side effects

Include nausea, headache, vomiting, diarrhea. Symlin is also associated with increased risk of insulin induced hypoglycemia.

Long Acting GLP-1

Long acting GLP-1 is taken once a week.

Bydureon

Bydureon releases the medication slowly and consistently over time. With each weekly dose, the amount of medicine in your body builds up until it reaches an optimal level after ten weeks, giving consistent control of glucose seven days a week.

Possible Side Effects

The most common side effect of bydureon is a bump at the injection site and nausea. Other side effects which are less common include headache, diarrhea, injection site redness, itching, and constipation.

Ozempic (Semaglutide)

Ozempic is also a long acting GLP-1 to be taken once a week.

Possible Side Effects

Nausea, vomiting, diarrhea, abdominal pain, and bloating

Trulicity (Dulaglutide)

Trulicity is another form of long acting GLP-1 which is to be taken once weekly.

Possible Side Effects

Most common side effects are nausea, vomiting, diarrhea, abdominal pain, and decreased appetite. Other side effects include pancreatitis and vision problems.

All GLP-1 agents have a black box warning for Medullary cancer of thyroid. GLP-1 has shown to be associated with a rare type of thyroid cancer called Medullary thyroid cancer in rodents. It has not shown to cause cancer in humans; however, GLP-1 agents should not be used if you have a personal or family history of Medullary thyroid cancer or Multiple Endocrine Neoplasia Type 2.

ORAL DIABETES MEDICATIONS

DRUG CLASS	HOW IT WORKS	SIDE EFFECTS
Biguanides Metformin/ Glucophage Fortamet Riomet	Increase insulin sensitivity Decrease amount of glucose released by the liver in between meals	Diarrhea most common Nausea, headache, metallic taste, lactic acidosis
Sulfonylureas Glyburide (Diabeta) Glipizide (Glucotrol)) Glimepiride (Amaryl)	Stimulates pancreas to release more insulin	Low blood glucose Weight gain
Meglitinides Repaglinide Nateglinide	Stimulates pancreas to make more insulin	Low blood glucose Weight gain
DPP-4 Inhibitors Sitagliptin (Januvia) Linagliptin (Tradjenta) Saxagliptin (Onglyza) Alogliptin (Nesina)	Inhibits the enzyme DPP-4 which inactivates GLP-1, Prolongs the action of GLP-1, which releases more insulin if BG is high after meal.	Upper respiratory tract infection, sore throat Stuffy nose Headache Joint pain Increase risk of pancreatitis
SGLT-2 Inhibitors Canagliflozin (Invokana) Empagliflozin (Jardiance) Dapagliflozin (Farxiga)	Lowers blood glucose by increasing the excretion of glucose in urine	Yeast infection Urinary tract infection Diabetic ketoacidosis
Thiazolidinediones Rosiglitazone (Avandia) Pioglitazone (Actos)	Makes tissue more sensitive to insulin	Weight gain Fluid retention Increase risk of fractures Liver problems Worsening heart failure

GLP-1 Agonist Rybelsus (Semaglutide)	Stimulates insulin secretion Lowers glucagon secretion when glucose is high Delays gastric emptying	Pancreatitis Hypoglycemia Acute kidney injury Diabetic retinopathy
Alpha glucosidase inhibitors Acarbose (Precose) Miglitol (Glyset)	Decreases the absorption of glucose form the gut	Nausea Bloating Gas
Dopamine agonist Bromocriptine (Cycloset)	Works centrally in the brain	Decreased BP Dizziness
Bile acid sequestrants Colveselam (Welchol)	Not known	Nausea Indigestion Gas

INSULIN

Insulin is a naturally occurring hormone in the body. It is secreted by the beta cells of the pancreas. For a person without diabetes, the body produces insulin throughout the day and night. Some insulin is produced all the time, which is called basal insulin production, but additional insulin is produced as soon as a person eats to process the glucose taken with meals.

People with Type 2 diabetes are not deficient in insulin in the initial stages, but the insulin they make is not good quality. They still have some insulin functioning and therefore, most Type 2 diabetics do not need insulin upon diagnosis as long as their glucose is not very high. As diabetes progresses, the beta cells in the pancreas burn out; that is when Type 2 diabetics need insulin. In some cases, the glucose level is very high upon diagnosis, and the person is in a state of glucose toxicity. In that case, insulin treatment is used initially to treat glucose toxicity, and when glucose levels come down to a reasonable level, then the person is switched to the oral or other injectable medications. In the past, insulin treatment was used as the last resort after all other diabetic medications failed; therefore, it was perceived by many as a punishment for not controlling glucose. However, research has shown that intensive insulin treatment of diabetes early on prevents long-term complications. Therefore, intensive treatment with insulin is sometimes the first course of action. Also, when you start with insulin, you are actually giving your cells in the pancreas a rest, thereby preserving them. Insulin is also the only drug that can be taken at any stage of kidney disease and heart disease; thus, if you have cardiovascular disease or kidney issues, insulin might be the only medication that is appropriate for you to use.

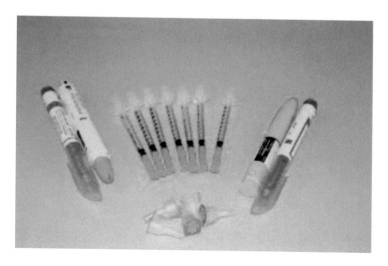

TYPES OF INSULIN.

Based on their duration of action insulins can be broadly classified into three different types:

- Basal Insulin (long acting)
- Intermediate acting Insulin
- Bolus Insulin (short acting)

BASAL INSULIN

Basal insulin is the long acting insulin. This insulin may last in your body from 24 to 48 hours. It does not peak and, therefore, has a relatively decreased risk of hypoglycemia.

Bolus or prandial insulin is the short acting insulin that is taken with meals to cover for the glucose from the food. This insulin starts working within 15-20 minutes and disappears in 4 to 6 hours therefore, it has to be taken multiple times with each meal during the day.

There are several different types of basal insulin

- Insulin Glargine (Lantus) action lasts 24 hours
- Insulin Glargine (Basaglar) action lasts 24 hours
- Insulin Detemir (Levemir) action lasts 12 hours
- Insulin Degludec (Tresiba) action lasts 36 hours

Concentrated Forms

Insulin Glargine and Degludec are also available in more concentrated forms. These forms are used for people on higher doses of insulin as less volume of insulin is administered for a given dose.

- Insulin Glargine U300 (Toujeo)
- Insulin Degludec U200(Tresiba)

BOLUS INSULIN OR SHORT ACTING INSULIN

- Humolog
- Novolog
- Apidra
- Fiasp
- Regular insulin
- Regular insulin U500 (Concentrated insulin)
- Afrezza (inhaled insulin)

Short acting insulin is also called Bolus insulin or Prandial insulin. Insulin analogs starts working within 15 minutes after administration and action lasts for about 4 to 6 hours. Therefore, it has to be taken before meals. The regular insulin starts working in about 30 minutes and lasts for about 6 to 8 hours and is associated with relatively higher risk of hypoglycemia compared to other insulin analogs.

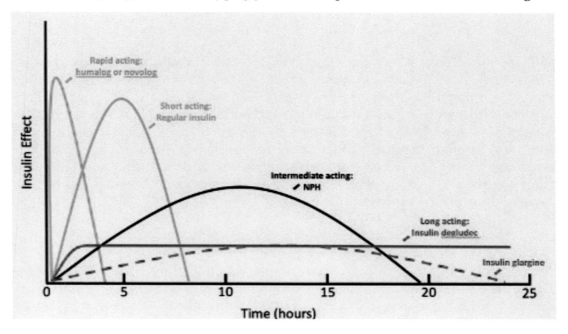

INHALED INSULIN (Afrezza)

Another form of short acting insulin is Afrezza which is an inhaled insulin. Afrezza has a very fast onset. Its glucose lowering action peaks in 12 minutes and stops after 1.5-2 hours. Afrezza 1.5 units is equal to 1 unit of injectable insulin. Afrezza is only available in 4 unit ampules, which is equivalent to 2.5 units of injectable insulin. Dose adjustment may be difficult for people on low doses of insulin or for those who require smaller increments

Afrezza should not be used by those who smoke and for people with chronic lung disease like asthma and COPD. Pulmonary function monitoring is required prior to starting Afrezza and periodically while on Afrezza.

INTERMEDIATE ACTING INSULIN

- NPH
- Humulin N
- Novolin N

Insulin NPH's onset of action is 2-4 hours, peaks in 4-10 hours and duration of action is 12-18 hours. It does not last a full 24 hours and, therefore, has to be taken twice a day. Unlike basal insulin, it has a peak and carries higher risk of hypoglycemia. Since Basal insulin does not have a peak, it lasts longer and, therefore, has a more stable glucose coverage. Use of NPH has considerably declined over the last decade.

PREMIXED INSULIN

NPH insulin also comes in combination with regular insulin as premixed insulin. It is available in different combinations like 70/30 where 70% is intermediate acting insulin and 30% is short acting insulin, and 70/25 where 70% is immediate intermediate acting insulin and 25% is short acting insulin. This type of insulin is used in some cases where the patient cannot take multiple injections and needs a simplified regimen. This type of insulin is not the best option, since it is a combination of two different types of insulin and each one will peak at a different time and may overlap. It carries a high risk of hypoglycemia and there is decreased flexibility for dose adjustment.

CONCENTRATED INSULIN (INSULIN HUMAN U500)

Insulin U500 is 5 times stronger than regular U100 insulin. It is specifically for people who are using over 200 units of regular insulin daily. U500 is a different kind of insulin compared to standard U100 insulin as it covers both long acting and mealtime needs. It is usually taken 2-3 times a day.

U500 can be delivered via U-500 Kwik Pen or using a special U500 syringe. It is important to only use the U500 syringe to inject U500 insulin as using a wrong syringe may result in delivering an incorrect dose of insulin.

Insulin U500 may cause severe hypoglycemic reaction if used incorrectly. Regular monitoring of blood glucose is extremely important when using U500 insulin.

Insulin U500 should not be used during pregnancy.

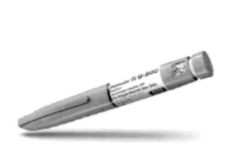
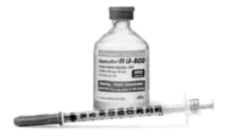

MULTIPLE DOSE INSULIN REGIMEN

The best way to take insulin is to match how insulin is naturally secreted in the body. When multiple injections of insulin are needed, the best way to take it is basal bolus regimen, which means you take a basal insulin that will last for 24 hours or more and take a bolus or short acting insulin before each meal to cover for your meals. Most often, using basal insulin by itself along with oral medications is enough. Mealtime insulin is often added later if needed.

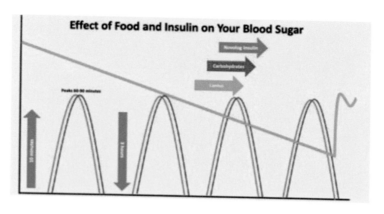

INJECTING INSULIN

Insulin can be injected using syringes or pens. Whether you choose to use syringes or pens depends on personal preference and insurance coverage and cost. Insulin syringes have been used for a long time. With syringes, one has to draw the desired amount of insulin from the vial. Syringes can hold a variety of insulin doses. Depending on what you are taking, you choose the size of the syringe. After taking the injection, the syringe has to be disposed of properly. Although not difficult, proper training is needed prior to using the syringes

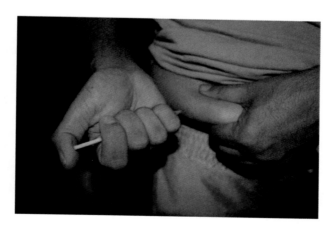

Insulin Pen

Insulin pens are more convenient and easier to use as they are prefilled with insulin and have a dial to adjust the amount of insulin to be taken when injected. A new pen needle has to be used with each dose of insulin and then disposed of. Insulin can be injected to any area of the body where there is fatty tissue. Absorption is best when injected in the abdomen, but it can also be injected in the thigh and the back of the arms. It is important to rotate the sites to avoid injection site problems such as infections and scar tissue development.

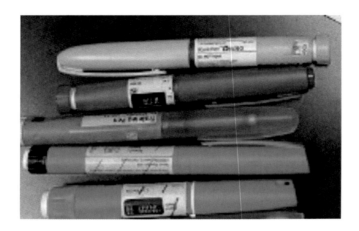

INSULIN PUMPS

An insulin pump is a device that can continuously deliver insulin in the body. An insulin pump consists of three parts: the tubing, the sensor, and the infusion sets. The pump is like a small computer that is programmed to deliver a certain amount of insulin into the body through a thin infusion set. The sensor is inserted under the skin with the needle that is removed, leaving a small catheter behind. The infusion set needs to be changed every 3 days for most pumps.

MINIMED™ 670G SYSTEM

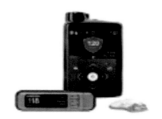

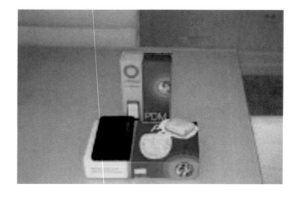

Insulin pumps use fast acting insulin. Insulin pumps can be worn at various regions of your body such as abdomen, back, gluteal region, hip, or thigh. People choose insulin pumps mainly due to flexibility of taking insulin. Some of the latest insulin pumps are connected with continuous glucose monitors which then talks to the pump and directly provide information on how much insulin to dispense. You still have to enter the amount of carbs taken at the meals. In some of the latest pumps the basal rate is automatically adjusted in the pump based on glucose levels. This is called the hybrid closed loop system and it is close to having an artificial pancreas.

Insulin pumps can offer great flexibility in terms of taking insulin; however, they are not easy for everyone to use. Proper training is required to understand various functions of the pump and adjust settings. It is important to understand the mechanics of the pump for troubleshooting. Proper carb counting training is also required before using the pump to be able to count the carbs correctly and put that information in the pump for the pump to calculate the insulin dose.

Indications for Insulin Pump

- Uncontrolled diabetes
- Frequent hyperglycemic excursions
- Frequent hypoglycemic reactions
- Hypoglycemic unawareness
- Unpredictable schedule
- Busy lifestyle
- Preconception
- Gestational diabetes
- People with diabetic gastroparesis

Who are Appropriate Insulin Pump Candidates?

- Patients who can monitor glucose with each meal
- Patients who are motivated and able to understand and handle the pump
- Patients willing to learn carb counting and implement it in their daily routine
- Patients willing to receive pump training
- Patients with a good support system

TYPES OF INSULIN

TYPE OF INSULIN	ONSET	PEAK	DURATION OF ACTION
Basal insulins Glargine (Lantus) Glargine (Basaglar) Glargine U300 (Toujeo) Detemir (Levemir) Degludec (Tresiba) Degludec U200 (Tresiba)	2-4 hrs 3-8 hrs 1 hour	No peak	20-24 hours 6-24 hours < 42 hours
Bolus insulins Humolog Novolog Apidra Fiasp Regular Regular U500 insulin Afrezza (Inhaled insulin)	5-15 min 2-5 min 30-60 min 5-10 min	60 min 30-90 min 2-3 hours 2-4 hours 12 min	3-5 hours 5 hours 5-8 hours 5-7 hours 1.5-2 hours
Intermediate acting insulin NPH	2-4 hours	4-10 hours	10-16 hours
Premix Insulin Intermediate + short	Combo NPH or reg 70%nph+30% reg 50%nph+ 50% reg	Dual peak	10-16 hours
Intermediate + rapid	Novolog mix- 70/30 Humolog mix- 70/25		

Chapter 7

WEIGHT MANAGEMENT

Being obese or overweight is the biggest risk factor for Type 2 diabetes. Obesity occurs due to a combination of genetic and environmental factors. This does not mean that if you have a genetic predisposition to obesity, you will be obese. We've seen that people today are much heavier than a few decades ago, which proves that environmental factors play a bigger role in development of obesity. This also proves that one can prevent being overweight or obese despite genetic preponderance by modifying their lifestyle and environment.

Most patients who develop Type 2 diabetes are overweight. Losing weight is extremely important and beneficial for Type 2 diabetes for various reasons. Excess fat in the body makes the cells resistant to the action of insulin and prevents glucose from entering the cell. As a result, the glucose remains in your blood, causing high blood glucose levels. The good news is that this process is reversible. As you lose weight, the cells become more sensitive to insulin again, allowing the glucose to enter the cells. Research has shown that losing as little as 7% of the body weight can have a significant impact on lowering glucose levels and preventing diabetes complications. As an added benefit, weight loss will make you look better and feel better about yourself.

To lose weight, you must take fewer calories in than calories out, which means you either eat less or burn more calories. This sounds straightforward, but it can be very challenging. It would be best to incorporate both diet (limiting calories) and physical activity (burning calories) into your lifestyle, but before you do that, it is important to have the correct mindset. Behavior modification and changing habits is the key to success in any weight-loss program. Several diets or weight-loss programs are out there, some of which are not appropriate for diabetics. You must always consider consulting your doctor before starting a new weight-loss program or diet. As much as you want to get the benefit from the diet, you also want to make sure it will not hurt you.

Before you choose a diet, you want to assess your goals and your readiness. Some of the questions to ask yourself would be:

- Are you overweight or obese?
- What is your waist circumference and current BMI?
- Is your goal to lose weight or to maintain your weight?
- Are you trying to lose weight due to health conditions?
- What are your restrictions?
- Do you have health conditions?
- Have you gained weight acutely or over a length of time?

BMI

BMI stands for body mass index. It is a calculation based on your height and weight to determine if you have an excess amount of fat in your body. It is commonly used to classify underweight, overweight, and obesity in adults. BMI is defined as the weight in kilogram divided by the height in meters squared (kg/m^2). One can calculate a BMI using a BMI chart or a BMI calculator.

WHO BMI Classification

Underweight	< 18.5
Normal weight	18.5 - 24.9
Overweight	25.0- 29.9
Obese	30.0 - 39.9
Morbid obese	> 40.0

BMI was developed as a risk indicator of disease. As BMI increases, the risk of certain diseases like diabetes and heart disease increases. It is very easy to calculate BMI using the BMI chart; however, like any other measure, it is not perfect as it is only dependent on height and weight and does not take into consideration different levels of adiposity based on age, physical activity, and sex. It is expected that it overestimates adiposity in some cases and underestimates in others.

BMI calculation can vary slightly in certain ethnic populations. For example, Asians have 2-5% higher total body fat. South Asians, in particular, are more prone to develop abdominal obesity which may account for a high risk of Type 2 diabetes. In Asians, normal BMI ranges between 18.5 to 22.9, Having a BMI of 23 is considered overweight, and a BMI of 27 is consistent with obesity.

WAIST CIRCUMFERENCE

Other measures such as waist circumference can complement BMI estimates. Waist circumference is a measure taken around the abdomen at the level of the umbilicus (belly button). A waist circumference over 40 in men and over 35 in women is associated with health problems such as increased risk of Type 2 diabetes, high cholesterol, high BP, and heart disease. In Asians, waist circumference cut off is 35.5 inches for men and 31.5 inches for women.

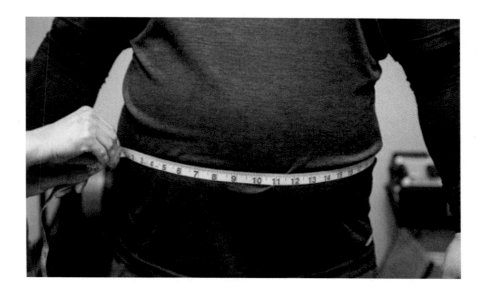

GOAL SETTING

Once you have determined your current weight status, the next step is goal setting. It is important to set up goals that are realistic and achievable. Setting unrealistic goals can only lead to frustration and disappointment.

You must have a long-term goal of what you want to achieve as an end point and a short-term goal that you would focus on daily to ultimately reach your long-term goal. Short-term goals must focus on not only the amount of weight you want to lose in a given time but also tracking the activities you are planning to do daily to achieve those goals such as changes in your diet and amount of physical activity. Writing down your goals and making a list of changes you are planning to make in your diet and activity to achieve your goal is very helpful, as you can keep track of your progress and see what works for you and what does not. If your current plan is not working, then you may have to reassess and adjust your goals and activity.

TIPS FOR SETTING WEIGHT-LOSS GOALS

- Set realistic goals
- Pick a goal that is practical for you to achieve at your given stage of life
- Set goals that suit your lifestyle
- Involve a diabetes educator or a dietitian
- Have a plan on how well you achieve your goal and how to track it

In general, setting up short-term goals to lose 1-2 pounds per week is healthy and achievable. If you add that up, it translates to about 52-104 pounds per year.

Research has shown that no one diet is superior to another. The American Diabetes Association does not recommend any specific diet program. A well-balanced diet with low carbs and low calories with regular physical activity is the one that works best for diabetics. However, the amount of carbohydrate restriction and calorie restriction may vary from person to person, depending on their current weight and blood glucose level.

Normal adult females ages 18-50 need approximately 1,800-2,000 calorie to maintain weight; normal adult males need approximately 2,400-2,800 calories to maintain weight. Those who have a sedentary lifestyle needs less calories than those more active. As a general rule, to lose one pound per week, you'll have to cut back at least 500 calories per day from your current calorie intake.

ACTIVITY LEVELS

Sedentary lifestyle means no additional activity other than activities of independent living. Moderate activity involves walking 3 miles per day or equivalent in addition to activities of independent living. Active lifestyle means doing activity that is equivalent to walking more than 3-4 miles per day.

Here is an example of an 1800 calorie meal plan:

SAMPLE MEAL PLAN

1800 Calories				
Meal	Exchange	Carb Grams	Food	Amount
Breakfast (60 gm carb)	2 starch 1 milk 1 fruit 1 fat	30 15 15 0	Bagel Skim.1% milk Banana Cream cheese, lite	1 medium 8 ounces 1 small 2 tablespoons
Lunch (60 gm carb)	2 starch 3 meat, 1 fat 1 veg (free) 1 fruit 1 milk	30 0 0 15 15	Whole grain bread Tuna salad (low fat) Raw veggies Strawberries Yogurt, lite	2 slices ¾ cup 1 cup 1 ¼ cup 6 ounces
Dinner (60 gm carb)	2 starch 1 starch 3 meats 1 veg (free) 1 veg (free) 1 fruit 1 fat	30 15 0 0 0 15 0	Pasta French bread Meatballs Marinara sauce Broccoli Canned pears Margarine, lite	1 cup 1 slice 3 golf ball sized ½ cup ½ cup cooked ½ cup 2 Tablespoons
Snack (30 gm carb)	1 starch 1 veg (free) 1 fruit	15 0 15	Baked tortilla Chips Salsa Orange	15 ½ cup 1 medium

Tips to combine weight loss with a healthy balanced meal plan:

- Have a consistent meal schedule
- Do not skip meals
- Maintain a diet and activity log
- Remove unhealthy snacks from your pantry and replace with healthy ones
- Make fruits and vegetables available and put them in visible spots so they are easy to grab
- Make water your preferred drink
- Add fresh fruit slices to water to add flavor instead of using juices
- Avoid eating while watching TV, as it may lead to overeating
- Try to distract yourself when you are craving an unhealthy snack by going out for a walk or calling a friend
- Ask a family member to try your meals and involve them in your diet
- Consider forming a group with friends or family to share your diet plan

TRACKING YOUR PROGRESS

Losing weight is not something that happens overnight. Planning ahead and keeping track of all the activities you are doing to lose weight is as important as the activity itself.

- After you have set up a carbohydrate and calorie goal for yourself, consider planning your meal for the next week
- If you're preparing your own meals, consider looking at the meal plan for the next day the night before to make sure you have all the ingredients for your cooking that day
- Weigh yourself once a week. Spend a few minutes every Sunday to tract your progress. Are you achieving your set goal for that week? If not, think about what got you off track and what you would do differently next time

COMMITMENT PARTNER

Having a commitment partner is another good way to stay on track and keep your self-motivated. Ask a friend or family member who wants to lose weight to become your commitment partner. Discuss your meal planned for the day with your partner the night before and ask each other if you followed your diet at the end of the day before you discuss the next day's meal. This is especially helpful if your partner is sharing the same meal plan as you, but it can be different. Also, your commitment partner does not have to have the same weight-loss goals as you.

WEIGHT LOSS MEDICATIONS

Weight loss medications are advised to a select group of patients who are overweight or obese, have tried diet and exercise, but have not been able to achieve significant weight reduction. Your doctor may consider prescribing a weight loss medication for you if you meet one of the following criteria:

- Your body mass index is greater than 30
- Your body mass index is greater than 27 and you have serious health problems related to your weight such as diabetes or high blood pressure

As much as one may dream of a weight-loss pill that would work without diet and exercise, the truth is that none of these drugs work that way. People who are placed on weight-loss medication still have to continue with diet regimens and exercise as tolerated to get the desired benefit. Almost all weight-loss medications have some side effects and cannot be used long term. Weight-loss medications cannot be used if you are pregnant or breastfeeding. It is not recommended to be started in a woman who is planning pregnancy and for those in reproductive age have to be placed on a reliable form of contraception prior to starting weight-loss medication.

A pregnancy test is often recommended prior to starting any of these medications.

It is important to have a detailed discussion with your health care team before starting a weight-loss medication. Your doctor will consider your health history, possible side effects, and interactions with your current medications.

Duration of Treatment with Weight-Loss Medications

This depends of whether the drug helps you lose weight and if you have had any side effects. Most weight-loss medications are advised to be discontinued if you do not lose between 3-5 % of body weight in the first 12 weeks. Your doctor may prescribe a different weight-loss medication. After stopping weight-loss medication, most people will gain some weight back; however, adopting a healthy lifestyle and having a transition plan may limit this weight gain.

Most people will lose a maximum of 10% of their body weight on weight-loss medication, which may not sound like a lot, but experts stress that as little as 5-7% weight loss can make a big difference in decreasing your risk of developing an obesity related disease.

Currently, six FDA-approved weight-loss medications are used in the United States.

CURRENT FDA APPROVED MEDICATIONS FOR WEIGHT LOSS

- Adipex-P (Phentermine)
- Qsymia   (Phentermine/Topiramate)
- Lomaira   (Phentermine low dose)
- Contrave (Naltrexone HCL/Bupropion HCL)
- Saxenda   (Liraglutide)
- Belviq   (Lorcaserin)
- Xenical   (Orlistat)
- Alli   (Orlistat)

BARIATRIC SURGERY

Surgery for obesity is considered as a last resort after diet, exercise, medications, and psychotherapy have failed. A generally accepted criterion for surgical treatment is a BMI over 40 or a BMI over 35 in combination with other comorbid conditions like diabetes, high BP, and sleep apnea.

Even for surgical procedures, the process starts with aggressive dietary restriction and monitoring when a person is placed on a very low-calorie diet protocol with behavior modification for at least 3 months prior to surgery. Currently, several different types of surgical procedures are performed, some of which are simpler than others

Gastric Bypass

Gastric bypass provides a considerable amount of dietary restriction, which is done by creating a small stomach pouch which then makes the person feel full after eating a small meal. This procedure, in addition to the restricting component, also decreases the absorption of nutrients from the gut. After a standard gastric bypass, a person can lose close to 100 pounds or about 60-70% of excess body weight.

After gastric bypass, some people may develop dumping syndrome upon ingestion of sweets. This occurs due to rapid passage of sugar directly to the intestine where presence of a big load of sugar causes abdominal pain and cramping. In addition, the rapid absorption of sugar triggers a rapid insulin response by the pancreas causing hypoglycemia. Eventually, these patients develop several vitamin deficiencies, requiring lifelong replacement and monitoring.

Gastric Sleeve Procedure

Sleeve gastrectomy involves removing a large portion of the stomach thus reducing the stomach size to 15-20% of the normal size. It also creates a restriction on the amount of food that can stay in the stomach and makes a person feel full after a small meal. However, this procedure does not cause the absorption problems that are seen with gastric bypass.

Laparoscopic Gastric Banding

In this procedure, an adjustable inflatable band is placed around the opening of the food pipe into the stomach. The smaller opening results in restriction of the amount of food that can pass into the stomach. After adjustable laparoscopic banding a person can lose up to 50-60% of excess body weight in 2 years.

There are many short-term and long-term complications associated with these surgical procedures and, therefore, the decision to get surgery for weight loss should be well thought out and discussed with a bariatric specialist with proper weighing of risks vs. benefits.

Chapter 8

WEIGHT LOSS PROGRAMS AND DIET PLANS

TYPES OF DIETS

We'll now review a variety of diet plans used for weight management. The American Diabetes Association does not recommend or endorse any specific diet for diabetes. Some of the diet plans may not be suitable for diabetics. A diabetic diet means a healthy balanced plate with small portions.

The idea of discussing the diets mentioned here is to give you a basic overview of the diets so you can make an informed decision if you choose to follow any of them. It is always advisable to talk to your doctor first before starting any diet or weight-loss program. Diet plans that will be discussed here are:

- Mediterranean diet
- Keto diet
- South Beach diet
- Adkins diet
- Paleo diet
- The Nutrisystem
- Weight Watchers
- Jenny Craig
- Intermittent fasting

MEDITERRANEAN DIET

Several small studies have been done to compare different diets, and no diet has proven to be superior to another except the Mediterranean diet, which has shown to reduce cardiovascular risk.

The Mediterranean diet is based on including healthy grains and herbs. It does not exclude any food group from the diet partially or completely. Mediterranean-style eating involves:

- Adding plenty of grains, beans, lentils, nuts, herbs, and spice
- Fish and seafood twice a week
- Use of healthy fats like olive oil
- Moderate amount of dairy
- Small amounts of red meat, saturated fat, and sugars

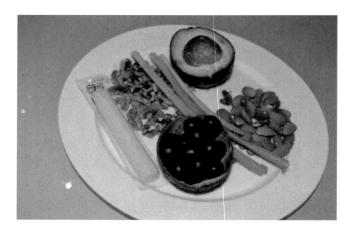

The Mediterranean diet has been there for hundreds of years and is the most researched diet. It has consistently demonstrated benefits in a long-term study of 26,000 healthy U.S. women published in 2018. In this study, risk of heart disease was reduced by 25% in those following the Mediterranean diet. Other studies done in Europe have shown similar results. The Mediterranean diet has also shown to be beneficial in reversing metabolic syndrome. Weight loss is more gradual, but health benefits are long term and more sustainable. Overall, the Mediterranean diet is considered safe to be used by children as well as by adults.

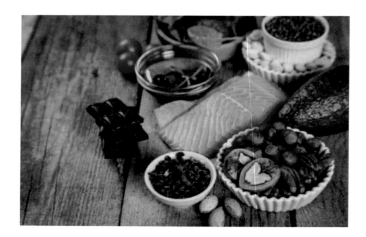

KETO DIET

The Keto diet is one of the most popular diets today, probably because of the ability to lose weight fast in a short time. There are many versions of Keto diet. Some will do it indefinitely, but others will cycle in and out. Keto diet emphasizes cutting back on carbs completely and, by doing so, going into a state of ketosis and use the fat for energy. The Keto diet is based on consuming high amounts of fat, which is burned for energy. Once in the state of ketosis, a person feels more energetic with improved mental focus, decreased hunger, change in exercise performance, and rapid weight loss.

Basics of Keto Diet

Keto plans involve restricting carbs to 15 to 20 carbs per day and obtaining 70% of calories from fat. Whole dairy foods are encouraged. Desserts like dark chocolate and peanut butter are allowed. For salads, green leafy vegetables like kale, spinach, broccoli, and lettuce are allowed, but starchy vegetables like corn and potato are not. Salad dressings can have oils like avocado, olive oil, canola, flaxseed, and palm oil or minerals. Some research has shown that Keto diet may help lower blood glucose levels, thus helping to prevent and control diabetes.

The Keto diet is also a high-fat diet, which increases the risk of heart disease. It may not be suitable for people with certain medical conditions, especially those with liver and gallbladder diseases. The use of the Keto diet by people on multiple insulin injections is controversial. The Keto diet can also cause electrolyte imbalance and constipation. It is best to discuss with your doctor before starting this diet.

Because keto is a restrictive diet, anyone who is dealing with an eating disorder should avoid the Keto diet. Children and women who are pregnant and nursing should also avoid Keto diet. Some modified versions of the Keto diet are similar but less extreme in its dependence on fat as the primary source of calories. In either case, a high-fat low-carb ratio can be challenging for people to achieve in daily life. It may be better to use Keto diet short-term to cut weight quickly or to cycle in and out rather than making it a lifestyle. The Keto diet was first discovered in 1920 as means of treating severe epilepsy in children. It was composed of 90% fat, 6% protein and 4% carb, which helped with epileptic seizures. It is still used today in people with seizures in whom other treatments have not been successful.

PALEO DIET

The Paleo diet is an elimination diet. It is based on the elimination of foods that were not eaten by paleolithic ancestors. Paleo philosophy believes that getting away from the eating and healthy habits that our ancestors practiced is contributing to the rise of chronic health problems. Paleo diet focuses on whole food, fruit, non-starchy vegetables, and plenty of meat. Beans, legumes, rice, grains, as well as dairy and alcohol are out. Paleo diet can be a good way to lose weight quickly by eliminating processed foods and carbohydrates. One drawback with the Paleo diet is that it eliminates grains, which greatly reduces fiber intake. This can lead to constipation and alter a person's gut biome. Adding lots of fatty red meat can also increase the risk of heart disease and certain forms of cancer.

SOUTH BEACH DIET

The South Beach diet is also a restrictive diet with two phases.

Phase 1

There is an initial 14-day restriction phase in which bread, pasta, baked goods, ice cream, alcohol, sugar, and fruits are all restricted. The idea of South Beach is somewhat similar to the Keto diet by eliminating sugar and getting the body in fat burning mode. The South Beach diet promises you will lose 10-13 pounds in the first 2 weeks by eliminating carbs and focuses on better cardiovascular health. The philosophy here's that by 2 weeks, you will correct how your body reacts to cravings for certain foods like sugar and how you can continue to eat healthy by making slight modifications.

Phase 2

After the initial 2 weeks, you will add back some carbohydrates but only good ones like brown rice and some fruits and vegetables. You can stay in this phase for a longer time as long as the weight-loss goal is achieved, one is expected to continue losing one to 2 pounds per week in phase 2, which is consistent with the recommendations from CDC about safe and sustainable weight loss.

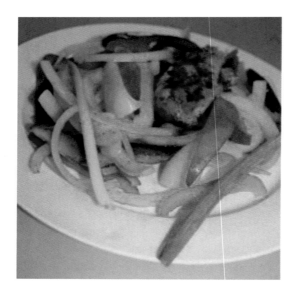

Maintenance Phase

Third and final phase is a more liberal maintenance phase for people who have achieved the desired weight-loss goal and are now trying to maintain the weight. This looks more like the Mediterranean diet with lots of fruits and vegetables, fresh lean meats, and dairy products.

Across all phases, the South Beach diet favors carbs with low glycemic index over high glycemic index. Low glycemic index carbs do not trigger an intense insulin response in the body and help you maintain steady blood glucose level.

ATKINS DIET

The Atkins diet is another low carb diet that was formed by cardiologists 40 years ago. It has four phases. You start by eating very low carbs and gradually increase as you reach your goal weight. The concept here is the same as the Keto diet; you use fat for fuel by avoiding carbohydrates, but you take more protein.

In phase one of Atkins, you take only 20% of carbs in your meal which is usually equivalent to 12 to 15 grams of carbs that come from vegetables, whereas you take 63% of fat. Atkins is comparable to keto in weight loss. Both are based on very low carbs intake, and both lower blood pressure and bad cholesterol.

NUTRISYSTEM

Nutrisystem is a weight-loss program founded in 1972. This system involves supplying prepackaged prepared meals and nutrition support to people seeking to lose weight.

Nutrisystem focuses on balanced nutrition and portion sizing. Glycemic index is the main focus of the program. As explained earlier, the glycemic index of a food determines how it affects the blood glucose levels. Food with similar content may have different glycemic index. Food with higher glycemic index will cause a much higher spike in glucose. Consumers will buy prepared meals but are encouraged to add fresh vegetables to the food. In addition, the company also provides nutritional counselors to the clients.

WEIGHT WATCHERS

Weight Watchers is the largest weight-loss program in the United States. It was founded in 1963. They rebranded in 2018, changing their focus from just weight loss to overall health and wellbeing.

Weight Watchers is a more flexible program and can be customized to individual needs. Weight Watchers has an assessment system that places the client into one of the three food plans, depending on their preference, activity levels, and desired goals. Every food or drink has an assigned point and members follow the plan using the point system. Members are given daily allowance for smart points plus some extra points weekly. Overall, the smart point system encourages the members to eat foods that are lower in calories, saturated fats, and sugar and higher in protein.

A delayed onset of diabetes was observed in one study in 2013 in those who did Weight Watchers for 10 months compared to standard diet. Weight Watchers offers gradual weight loss of one to 2 pounds per week and; therefore, it can be followed long term. Even though it is relatively safe, it is not recommended for children and pregnant females.

JENNY CRAIG

Jenny Craig is a weight-loss program based on restriction of total calories, fat, and portion sizing. This plan also requires clients to enroll in a program that provides packaged meals and snacks along with personalized counseling. In the Jenny Craig system, you have six meals a day, three meals, two snacks, and a dessert. Clients do not have to count calories or measure portions while on the program. Counseling sessions are via face-to-face appointments, web-based appointments, or phone calls. The program works best for people who do not have time to shop or cook or count calories. Jenny Craig is not a good option for people on a gluten-free diet, as most of their meal plans contain gluten ingredients.

INTERMITTENT FASTING

Intermittent fasting involves voluntary abstinence from food and drink. Fasting is an ancient practice followed in a variety of different formats all over the world.

How Intermittent Fasting can Help you with Weight Loss

The food we eat is broken down into simple sugars by enzymes in your stomach and eventually ends up in your bloodstream from where it is taken into your cells. If the cells do not use the sugar for energy then it is stored in the form of fat, but as we discussed in an earlier chapter, that sugar needs insulin to enter the cells. Between meals, if we do not snack, then our insulin levels will go down and our fat cells can then release stored sugar, which is used as energy.

The idea of fasting is based on the fact that when we allow our insulin levels to go down far enough, we start burning fat for energy. There is good evidence that fasting, when combined with a healthy diet, can be an effective approach to weight loss. Fasting is associated with lower insulin levels, increased insulin sensitivity, improved metabolism, lower cholesterol levels, lower blood sugar, and less inflammation. A variety of different forms have been used for intermittent fasting, including daily intermittent fasting to alternate day fasting versus extended night time fasting, which involves having the last meal of the day around three pm and then fast until the next morning. Research has shown that consuming most of the energy earlier in the day, thus increasing the time in the evening and the night when no food is consumed is associated with weight loss and improved health outcomes. However, it appears that almost any intermittent fasting regimen can result in some weight loss. Overall, intermittent fasting does not cause any harm physically or mentally. However, it must be used cautiously when people are taking multiple medications throughout the day. Diabetics may need adjustment in the medications if following intermittent fasting, especially if they're using insulin. It is recommended that people with advanced diabetes, eating disorders, and breastfeeding or pregnant females should not attempt intermittent fasting.

Chapter 9

COMPLICATIONS OF DIABETES

Diabetes is a chronic disease. One can lead a completely normal life with diabetes as long as blood glucose is well controlled. However, uncontrolled diabetes can lead to serious health problems. Diabetes complications can be acute or chronic. Acute complications occur due to a sudden increase in glucose levels, often due to an illness or noncompliance with medications. Chronic or long-term complications are caused by years of uncontrolled high blood glucose levels. In this chapter, we'll describe the acute and chronic complications of diabetes and how we can effectively manage them.

ACUTE COMPLICATIONS OF DIABETES

Acute complications of diabetes are those that arise quickly from uncontrolled blood glucose or from low blood glucose. They are serious and may be life threatening and require immediate attention. Such complications, if treated appropriately and promptly, can go away as fast as they occur. Three most important acute complications of diabetes that requires immediate attention are:

- Diabetic ketoacidosis
- Diabetic non ketotic hyperosmolar state
- Hyperglycemia
- Hypoglycemia

DIABETIC KETOACIDOSIS (DKA)

Diabetic ketoacidosis is a condition caused by inadequate insulin. It is more common in Type 1 diabetes but can also occur in Type 2 diabetes.

Causes of DKA in Type 2 Diabetes

- Newly diagnosed or unknown diabetes
- Another medical condition that will raise blood glucose such as infection
- If one stops taking medication abruptly
- High blood glucose due to steroid treatment

What Happens in DKA?

Without insulin, the body cannot use glucose and it is stored as fat. As a result, the fat comes out of the cells and goes to the liver where it is converted to glucose and keto acids, also known as ketones. These levels build up in the blood causing diabetic ketoacidosis.

Signs and Symptoms of DKA

Nausea, vomiting, abdominal pain, fruity breath, frequent urination, increased thirst, blurred vision, weakness, fatigue, heavy breathing, confusion, and coma.

What to do?

Check your ketones if your glucose is over 250 or if you are feeling sick or stressed, even if your glucose is lower. Ketone test kits are available in all pharmacies. Kits have certain chemical treated strips that you dip into your urine. The strip would change color according to the level of ketones in your urine. If the color in the test strip shows moderate or high ketones, or if your glucose is high and you are feeling sick, you must call your doctor or go to emergency for evaluation. Diabetic ketoacidosis is associated with moderate to severe electrolyte imbalance. It requires immediate attention.

Treatment

DKA is usually treated with aggressive IV hydration. Insulin is frequently given in the form of continuous drip until the body stops making ketones. Electrolytes are monitored every 4-6 hours and replaced as needed. Gradually the blood glucose comes to normal and the body stops making ketones. Adjusting blood glucose too quickly can sometimes lead to swelling in the brain and therefore diabetic ketoacidosis is treated over a period of 12 to 24 hours. If left untreated DKA can lead to coma and possible death.

DIABETIC NONKETOTIC HYPEROSMOLAR STATE (HHS)

This is more common in Type 2 diabetes. It is a life-threatening emergency with very high blood glucose levels, usually over 600. Unlike diabetic ketoacidosis, diabetic hyperosmolar state develops over time and often occurs due to another medical problem such as dehydration, infection, stress, heart attack, or stroke. Not drinking enough water is one of the most common reasons for hyperosmolar state.

This is especially true for nursing homes and the elderly who do not have access to free fluids or do not want to drink so they do not have to go to the bathroom. The elderly also frequently forget to drink water.

In diabetic hyperosmolar state, the body tries to dispose of excess sugar in the urine. The urine gets concentrated and pulls fluid from the body and more water is lost leading to severe dehydration. If this condition continues, severe dehydration can lead to confusion, seizures, or coma.

Signs and Symptoms of HHS

- Glucose is usually over 350 mg/dl
- Increase frequency of urination
- Extreme thirst
- Dry mouth
- Warm, dry skin
- High fever
- Confusion
- Drowsiness
- Weakness
- Stupor
- Coma

What to do?

Since the hyperosmolar state develops over time, you have a window of opportunity to prevent it from worsening. Drink plenty of fluids if you are sick. Call your doctor if you have signs and symptoms of dehydration or if blood glucose is very high.

Treatment

- Hospitalization
- Aggressive IV fluids
- Insulin treatment
- Electrolyte monitoring and replacement
- Close monitoring

HYPERGLYCEMIA

Hyperglycemia is defined as glucose level that is higher than normal. Having persistently high glucose levels can lead to complications. Hyperglycemia does not cause any symptoms initially, and is therefore frequently not addressed until it gets too bad. When blood glucose goes higher, it can cause symptoms of fatigue, lack of energy, increased frequency of urination, increased thirst, dry and itchy skin, and blurred vision. The only way to track hyperglycemia early on is to monitor your glucose regularly and if it is higher than normal, talk to your doctor, as you may need adjustment in your medication.

Dawn Phenomenon

Dawn Phenomenon is the recurrence of elevated blood glucose during early morning hours roughly between 4-8 am. It is thought to be due to the effect of other hormones such as adrenaline, cortisol, glucagon, and growth hormone which are found in higher concentrations in the blood in the morning and promote glucose release into the blood.

The processes of dawn phenomenon occur in everyone regardless of whether they have diabetes or not. The difference lies in how our bodies react to it. Healthy individuals secrete enough insulin and are insulin sensitive enough to counteract a rise in morning blood glucose. However, someone with prediabetes or Type 2 diabetes is insulin resistant and may not secrete enough insulin, which allows blood glucose to rise. This is further compounded by the fact that in the early morning hours our body is more insulin resistant compared to the rest of the day.

CHRONIC COMPLICATIONS OF DIABETES

Chronic or long-term complications of diabetes develop gradually and occurs due to damage to your blood vessels from persistent high blood glucose. Blood vessels are your transport system to carry essential nutrients and oxygen to your brain, heart, kidneys, and other vital organs. When these blood vessels are damaged, blood supply to vital organs is decreased, leading to complications. You can keep your blood vessels healthy by keeping your blood glucose, blood pressure, and cholesterol in good shape. This means eating healthy food with less sugar, fat, and cholesterol, exercising regularly, losing weight, and not smoking. The good news is that these complications can be delayed or completely prevented by keeping your blood vessels healthy.

Most complications develop without causing any symptoms in the initial stage. It is therefore important to get regular screening for these complications. Diabetes affects almost every organ system in the body. Some systems are affected more than the others. We will now discuss each complication individually to get a better understanding of what diabetes does and how you can prevent it.

HEART DISEASE

Diabetes is called a coronary artery disease equivalent, which means if you have diabetes, you are at the same risk of having a heart attack as someone who already had one. Risk of heart disease in diabetes is 2-4 times higher than in the normal population. Diabetes can damage major arteries carrying blood supply to your heart by making them prone to fatty deposits, causing blockages and hardening. This condition is called atherosclerosis.

occurs in everyone

Coronary Artery Disease

Coronary arteries are the blood vessels that carry blood supply and oxygen to the heart. Coronary artery disease is caused by blockage in these blood vessels. Because of these blockages there is less oxygen supply to the heart muscle, leading to muscle damage

Signs and Symptoms of Coronary Artery Disease

- Chest pain
- Fatigue
- Shortness of breath
- Decreased exercise tolerance

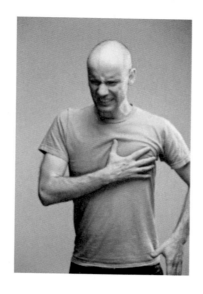

Signs and Symptoms of a Heart Attack

- Chest pressure
- Squeezing pain in the center of the chest
- Pain extending to the shoulders, arm, jaw, or back
- Shortness of breath
- Sweating
- Palpitations
- Lightheadedness
- Fainting
- Nausea

- Vomiting
- Impending sense of doom

If you suspect that you or someone else is having a heart attack, call 911 immediately, as the timing from having a heart attack to getting treatment is crucial. The longer you wait, the more heart damage occurs and chances of survival are significantly decreased.

Silent Heart Attack

It is important to note that diabetics may not have the typical signs and symptoms of having a heart attack due to nerve damage and, therefore, mild symptoms should not be ignored.

Heart Failure

People with diabetes are also at increased risk for having heart failure without a heart attack.

Tips for prevention of heart attack:

- Keep your blood glucose in good control
- Keep your blood pressure and cholesterol in good control
- Eat healthy
- Exercise regularly
- Quit smoking
- Take medications for your diabetes, blood pressure, and cholesterol regularly
- Do not miss your doses or stop medication abruptly

STROKE

A stroke is another major complication associated with diabetes. Stroke occurs when blood supply to your brain is blocked, resulting in decreased oxygen and nutrient supply to the brain. Brain cells can die within a few minutes to a few hours.

There are different types of strokes:

- **Ischemic Stroke** occurs when an artery supplying the brain is blocked
- **Hemorrhagic Stroke** occurs when an artery supplying the brain becomes leaky or ruptures

Signs and Symptoms of Stroke

- Numbness in the face or arm

- Facial drooping
- Weakness
- Paralysis of arm legs or one side of the body
- Speech difficulty
- Sudden blurred vision or decreased vision
- Dizziness
- Loss of balance
- Sudden worse headache
- Confusion
- Memory loss

TRANSIENT ISCHEMIC ATTACK

An early stroke can also present as transient ischemic attack which occurs when there is a transient block in the artery giving signs and symptoms that resolve as the blockage is resolved. This can last for a few minutes to a couple of days. Your doctor may not see any changes in your CT scan because of TIA, since by the time the imaging is done, the blockage usually resolves. However, TIA should be taken as a warning sign and complete evaluation should be done for assessment of risk.

Tips to Prevent Stroke

- Control your blood pressure
- Take appropriate medications
- Take TIA (Transient ischemic attack) seriously

MICROVASCULAR COMPLICATIONS

Microvascular complications of diabetes include neuropathy, nephropathy, and retinopathy.

NEUROPATHY

Nerve damage is a common complication of uncontrolled diabetes. Various systems in the body are connected to the brain via a network of nerves that carry messages back and forth between the body and the brain. High blood glucose can damage the tiny blood vessels supplying these nerves, resulting in nerve damage and symptoms of neuropathy. Symptoms depend on what nerve is damaged.

Damage to the sensory nerves will cause numbness and tingling starting in the fingers and toes. Loss of pain sensation makes you more prone to injury and infection. Stabbing pain at night and crawling sensation are also symptoms of neuropathy. Damage to autonomic nerves can lead to increased heart rate and perspiration. It can also lead to erectile dysfunction in men. Damage to nerves in the muscles may cause muscle weakness and loss of strength.

PERIPHERAL VASCULAR DISEASE

Peripheral vascular disease occurs due to buildup of plaque causing blockages in the peripheral vessels supplying your extremities especially your legs and feet. This is similar to what happens in the heart and brain. Decreased circulation in the legs and feet can cause leg cramps, difficulty walking, delayed wound healing, infection, and gangrene in some cases leading to amputation.

Screening for PVD

Your doctor can check the circulation in your extremities by doing a test called ankle brachial index. This test measures blood pressure in your upper arms and compares that with the blood pressure in your ankle. The difference in BP between your upper and lower extremities is suggestive of peripheral vascular disease.

How to Prevent PVD

- Stop smoking. Smoking makes peripheral vascular disease worse
- Exercise will help improve circulation
- Screen for PVD if symptoms are present

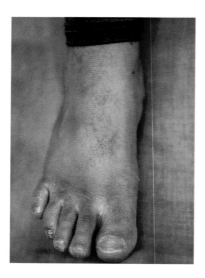

DIABETIC FOOT

Foot problems are common in diabetes due to a combined effect of nerve damage, decreased circulation, and increased risk of skin infections. A non-healing ulcer can progress to severe damage to tissues and gangrene, requiring amputation of a toe or the entire foot or leg. Over 80% of amputations begin with a simple foot ulcer and 5 out of 6 amputations performed are due to diabetes.

Charcot Joint

Charcot joint or diabetic neuropathic arthropathy is another common complication of diabetes. It occurs when a joint deteriorates because of nerve damage. It starts with numbness or tingling and loss of sensation in the affected joint. It then becomes warm, red, and swollen and unstable or deformed. It may not be very painful due to nerve damage. As the disease progresses, the joint gets weaker and starts losing calcium. Calcium is responsible for keeping the bones strong. With more and more calcium loss, the bones become weaker and break. Charcot joints can be treated, but it can take several months. You must see your doctor if you are experiencing any symptoms in your feet.

Foot Care

- Keeping your blood glucose in good control is the best way to prevent foot infection and delayed healing and other foot related complications
- Protect your feet from developing ulcers and treat any cuts immediately
- Visually check your feet every day
- Prevent excessive dryness and cracks in the feet that would break the skin
- All diabetics should get an annual foot exam by a healthcare provider to check for loss of sensation, ingrown toenails, cuts, blisters, ulcers, and fungus in the nails
- Wear comfortable shoes and socks
- Do not walk barefoot

NEPHROPATHY

Forty percent of the people with diabetes will have diabetic kidney damage. Kidneys are the clearing system of the body. When blood flows to the blood vessels in the kidneys, it filters out what our body needs and eliminates the rest of the waste in urine. High blood glucose as well as blood pressure can damage the small blood vessels in the kidney's filtering system, making them leaky. In early stages, the kidneys start leaking a protein called albumin. Albumin keeps the water in your blood vessels. When your kidneys start leaking, the albumin in the water is unable to stay inside and cause swelling in the ankles and feet and puffiness of the face. These are some of the early signs of kidney damage. Seven percent of diabetics already have some kidney damage at the time of diagnosis.

Screening for Diabetic Nephropathy

Kidney damage can be determined by a couple of different tests.

Urine Microalbumin Test

In this test, leakage is measured as milligrams of protein in your urine. Normally, the protein leakage should be less than 30 milligrams. A urine microalbumin level between 30 to 299 milligrams indicates early stage kidney damage. Urine microalbumin test is done once a year in a random urine sample to detect the presence of kidney damage.

Glomerular Filtration Rate (GFR)

Another test that can be done to check the level of kidney damage is glomerular filtration rate. GFR is part of the comprehensive panel that your doctor routinely orders. GFR slowly declines with age. However, uncontrolled diabetes can make this process happen much faster.

Many diabetic medications cannot be taken if your GFR is under a certain level. There is no fixed level. Different medications have different cut off levels for GFR. It is important to discuss this with your doctor when you are starting any new medication.

Protein leakage in the urine can also occur due to other reasons. Your doctor may have to do more testing to confirm that your kidney disease is secondary to your diabetes. If you have advanced kidney damage, you may be sent to see a kidney specialist (Nephrologist)

END STAGE KIDNEY DISEASE

End stage kidney disease or chronic kidney disease stage five occurs when your kidney stops working completely to a point that it cannot filter out the waste from your body. At this point, you may need to start dialysis to help your body filter out waste products.

What is Dialysis?

Dialysis is an artificial procedure to remove waste from your blood when your kidneys cannot do it. There are two types of dialysis procedures: hemodialysis and peritoneal dialysis.

Hemodialysis

A procedure in which blood is pumped out of your body through a fistula that is surgically created and connected to a machine that functions as an artificial kidney and filters out excess waste, extra fluids and returns the blood back to circulation.

Most patients need hemodialysis three times a week. This type of dialysis is usually done in a dialysis center. During hemodialysis, one may experience low blood glucose, cramps, or upset stomach. People on hemodialysis also need to be on a specific renal diet in addition to diabetic diet.

Peritoneal Dialysis

This is another form of dialysis that uses a network of tiny blood vessels in your abdomen to filter waste. A dialysis solution is infused into your abdomen and drained out to remove waste. Peritoneal dialysis can be done at home and allows more flexibility. Complications associated with peritoneal dialysis include infection, hernia, and weight gain.

Kidney Transplant

Kidney transplant is an alternate treatment for end stage kidney disease. It offers the best chance to restore normal kidney function and more regular lifespan and improve survival. However, for a transplant you have to match and you may have to be on the waiting list for a long time. Even with the best possible medicine, the immune system will try to reject the new kidney and, therefore, people with a kidney transplant have to go on several immunosuppressive medications for the rest of their lives.

The medications used in kidney transplant patients may have additional side effects. Therefore, it is important to make a thoughtful and well-informed decision prior to deciding on a kidney transplant. The best thing is to try to delay or prevent kidney damage altogether.

Tips for Preventing Kidney Damage

- Keep your blood glucose on target
- Keep your blood pressure on target
- Take recommended medications for blood pressure such as Angiotensin converting enzyme inhibitors and Angiotensin receptor blockers
- Get your routine screening for kidney damage once a year
- Eat foods low in sodium to control blood pressure

DIABETIC RETINOPATHY

Diabetic retinopathy is the leading cause of blindness in the United States in people aged 20-74 years. The American Diabetes Association recommends eye exam for all Type 2 diabetics by a specialist upon diagnosis and annually. Uncontrolled diabetes can damage small blood vessels supplying the eyes, leading to retinal damage. Often, no change in vision is noted in early retinopathy; therefore, the only way to find out is by a routine eye exam. Retinopathy can be easily treated if found in early stages. Diabetic retinopathy is of two types:

- Proliferative Retinopathy
- Nonproliferative Retinopathy

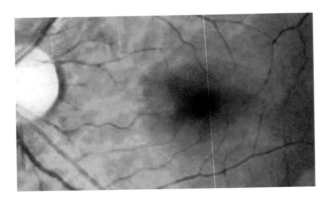

Nonproliferative Retinopathy

Nonproliferative retinopathy occurs in one in every five people. High blood glucose damages small blood vessels in the retina which bulge to form pockets called aneurysms. This makes the walls weak and leaky. Vision is not affected at this point. However, as damage progresses, blood vessels start leaking more and more fluid causing the retina to swell. When swelling involves the center of the retina called the macula, the vision starts getting affected. Nonproliferative retinopathy, if diagnosed early, can be completely treated.

Proliferative Retinopathy

Proliferative retinopathy is a less common and more severe form of retinopathy where the leaky blood vessels completely close and new blood vessels are formed that grow in the retina and affect vision. These new blood vessels are fragile and rupture, causing swelling and macular edema. The macula is the central part of the retina that helps you see fine details. Swelling of the macula is called macular edema. Once you have macular edema, it can cause blurred vision, decreased vision, and complete loss of vision.

Proliferative retinopathy can be treated with laser if found early. Lasers can patch up leaky blood vessels and destroy new blood vessels. Laser also discourages new vessel formation. More advanced retinopathy is treated with vitrectomy which is a procedure done to remove fluid from the eyes by making a small incision. Medications called VEGF (Vascular endothelial growth factors) are injected in some cases when the laser is not effective. These medications have promising results but are not used as standard of care.

Signs and Symptoms of Advanced Retinopathy

- Narrowed vision
- Floaters (Tiny specks and spiders floating in front of the eyes)
- Flashes of light
- Poor night vision
- A dark spot in the center of the vision
- Complete loss of vision

Two other eye conditions are very common in diabetics.

CATARACTS

Cataracts are common in the elderly but in diabetics, Cataracts can occur at a much younger age. Cataracts are a condition in which the lens becomes cloudy. It can be treated with surgery, during which the lens is replaced by a new plastic lens.

GLAUCOMA

Glaucoma is 40 times more common in diabetics than in non-diabetics. In glaucoma, there is increased pressure in the eyes, which causes fluid to build up and damage the retina and the optic. Glaucoma can also be treated with medications or surgery.

Tips to Prevent Retinopathy

- Control your blood glucose level with diet and exercise
- Control your blood pressure, quit smoking
- Get regular eye checkup
- Follow up as recommended by your eye doctor

Some people may need more frequent checkups and then annual visits. One must get immediate attention for any symptoms like blurred vision, black out, decreased night vision, and shadows.

GUM DISEASE (Dental Hygiene)

Dental hygiene is another important aspect of diabetic care, which is often ignored. Diabetics are recommended to go for a dental exam at least twice a year. Your Mouth harbors many bacteria. Since diabetics are more prone to infections, these bacteria can easily settle in your gums and cause infection. Some studies have also linked gum infection with cardiovascular disease, bacteria from the damaged gum enters the bloodstream and causes inflammation throughout the body, leading to plaque buildup, increasing the risk of heart attack and stroke.

How to Prevent Gum Disease

- Keep glucose in target range
- Clean your teeth well with regular brushing and flossing
- See your dentist at least twice a year for routine cleaning
- Look for signs and symptoms of gum damage like bleeding, swollen gums, and redness

DIABETIC GASTROPARESIS

Your digestive system is also affected by diabetes. Diabetes damages small blood vessels supplying the nerves in your gut. One of the nerves that may be damaged is the vagus nerve. The vagus nerve controls the movement of food through the stomach. Gastroparesis is a condition in which the movement of food through stomach and intestine slows down resulting in delayed gastric emptying.

Signs and Symptoms of Gastroparesis

- Bloating
- Nausea
- Vomiting
- Abdominal pain
- Loss of appetite
- Reflux and Weight loss
- Fluctuation in blood glucose

People with gastroparesis have frequent hyperglycemic and hypoglycemic excursions, which makes it difficult to manage diabetes. Gastroparesis can be diagnosed with the help of a barium meal test or gastric manometry.

Management of Gastroparesis

If you have gastroparesis, your doctor may advise you to monitor your glucose more frequently. You may need to adjust your medications. You may be given medications to stimulate your stomach muscle.

You may have to avoid drugs that slow down the gastric emptying such as opiates. You may need changes in your diet and eating habits. Patients with gastroparesis are recommended to have small, frequent meals instead of three large meals.

DIABETIC DERMOPATHY

Diabetic dermopathy is associated with long-term uncontrolled diabetes. These are Brown spots on the shins, which are thought to be due to damage to the small blood vessels resulting in leakage of blood products. Skin is the most important defense system in the body. High blood glucose can increase the risk of bacterial and fungal infections of the skin. Common bacterial infections seen frequently in diabetics are stye, boils, carbuncles, and furuncles. Furuncles are clusters of boils which may contain infected pus. Common fungal infections include athlete's foot, vaginal infections, nail infections. Most fungal infections occur in warm, moist, and dark places. People with diabetes also have dry peeling skin, especially in the feet. These can lead to cracks in the skin that can be a source of entry of bacteria into the body.

Tips to Prevent Skin Infections

- Keep your skin clean
- Hydrate your skin with moisturizer
- Drink plenty of water
- Protect your skin by using sunscreen

PSYCHIATRIC PROBLEMS

People with diabetes have several mental health issues, especially depression, anxiety, and dementia. Diabetics can have a combination of these disorders collectively called as diabetes distress.

What is Diabetes Distress?

Nearly half of diabetics suffer from diabetes distress. It is a state of feeling fear, anxiety, and frustration that comes with managing diabetes. The expectation for diabetics to maintain their glucose in good range, eat healthy, exercise, and take medications on time can sometimes be overwhelming, especially when they are also dealing with complications. Diabetes distress can have a major impact on one's ability to manage diabetes. Getting into therapy and talking to a physician at depth can help resolve some of the distress.

DEPRESSION

Like any other chronic illness, diabetes is strongly associated with depression. Untreated depression can have serious clinical implications. Routine depression screening is recommended for all diabetics.

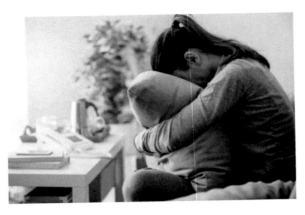

Coping with Stress

Stress can have a major impact on diabetes management. Stress not only raise your blood glucose level but also makes it harder to follow a healthy lifestyle. Stress can be of many kinds. It can be due to handling multiple medical problems, a family situation, a work-related issue, or sickness. Whatever it may be, you have to learn to manage stress in a positive way. For some people, it is difficult to speak about their needs to a spouse, another family member, work colleagues, or a provider.

Tips to Overcome Stress

- Learning to say no. For example, if you are expected to join a friend for an ice cream treat, something that you are not supposed to eat, do not be ashamed to politely say no
- Do not wait to eat until others eat, even if you think you must, as you might get hypoglycemic
- Practice deep breath several times during the day
- Activities like meditation and yoga are very helpful in destressing
- Consider joining a support group for diabetes
- Get enough sleep
- Talk to a therapist
- Do not hesitate to use medications if needed
- Educate your friends and family about diabetes. That way, they will understand what you are trying to achieve
- Strengthen your support system

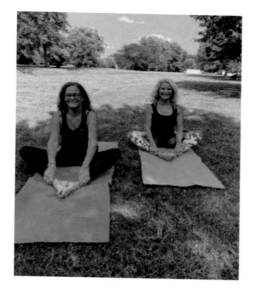

SKELETAL COMPLICATIONS OF DIABETES

Diabetes is also associated with various joint and bone problems.

Osteoporosis

People with diabetes are at increased risk of developing osteoporosis. The risk of osteoporosis is directly proportional to the duration of diabetes and level of control.

Frozen Shoulder

This is a condition that is frequently seen in diabetics. It's associated with pain, stiffness, and decreased range of motion.

Dupuytren's Contracture

This is the condition in which one or more fingers is bent towards the palm. It occurs with longstanding diabetes. It is caused by scarring of the connective tissue in the fingers and the palm.

Diffuse Idiopathic Skeletal Hyperostosis (DISH)

This is a condition characterized by hardening of the tendons and ligaments around the spine, resulting in stiffness and decreased range of motion. It is thought to be due to insulin and insulin growth factors that promote bone growth.

Chapter 10

DIABETES IN WOMEN

Women with diabetes face unique challenges due to hormonal fluctuation as well as other social factors. Studies have shown that blood sugar levels are more difficult to control in women compared to men. Women with diabetes have a sixfold higher risk of heart attack compared to men and they're more likely to die from a heart attack than men. Women are likely to have atypical presentations with heart attacks. Women with diabetes are also more likely to have chronic kidney disease as well as depression. Hormonal fluctuations make blood sugars more unpredictable in women. Better diabetes education and aggressive management can overcome these challenges.

MANAGING DIABETES DURING MENSES AND PREMENSTRUAL PHASE

Like their menstrual cycle, women's experience with managing diabetes during the menses differ. Women may notice erratic blood glucose right around her period or during the period. Interestingly, some women have frequent low glucose during menses and premenstrual period. By keeping a record of how the glucose trends are during menses for 2-3 consecutive months, you can determine the pattern and take action accordingly. For example, if you tend to have higher glucose during your menstruation, then you may have to adjust your insulin dose during your period every month. Adjustment in diet and meal timings may also help. If you get low reactions, you may want to take a couple of extra snacks or divide your meals into frequent small meals per day. You must discuss the management of glucose during menstrual and premenstrual phases with your health care provider.

PLANNING FOR PREGNANCY

Women with diabetes can have healthy pregnancies and babies as long as the blood glucose is well controlled during pregnancy. High blood glucose is associated with several complications during pregnancy and can be harmful for both mom and the baby. High glucose can increase the risk of the baby being larger, resulting in difficult and complicated delivery. Diabetes also increases the risk of preeclampsia, a condition usually occurring in the second or third trimester of pregnancy. It is characterized by high blood pressure, water retention, and weight gain. In severe cases, it may progress to eclampsia, increasing the risk of poor outcomes for both the mother and the baby. High blood glucose can pass on to the baby, resulting in birth defects and miscarriages. It is very important for a woman with diabetes to plan her pregnancy to make sure her blood glucose is in goal range before she gets pregnant.

GESTATIONAL DIABETES

Gestational diabetes is the diabetes that is diagnosed first time during pregnancy. All nondiabetic pregnant women are screened for gestational diabetes with a 75-gram oral glucose tolerance test between 24 to 28 weeks of pregnancy. This type of diabetes can be easily managed with diet in most cases. Some women may need to be treated with medication during gestational diabetes. For most of the cases, blood glucose will return to normal after pregnancy. Women with gestational diabetes are at increased risk of developing Type 2 diabetes within the next 5 years. Women with gestational diabetes have the same risk of maternal and fetal complications as women with Type 1 and Type 2 diabetes.

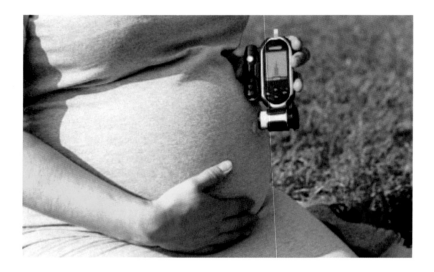

Glucose Monitoring During Gestational Diabetes

Women with gestational diabetes are advised to monitor glucose fasting and 1-2 hours after meals. The targets for blood glucose during pregnancy in women with gestational diabetes and Type 1 and Type 2 diabetes are slightly different and more aggressive.

Target glucose during pregnancy	
Fasting	< 95
One hour post prandial	<140
Two hours postprandial	<120

Management of Diabetes During Pregnancy

Management of diabetes during pregnancy can be very challenging. As highlighted before, gestational diabetes is associated with increased risk of birth defects and macrosomia. Treatment is associated with improved perinatal outcome.. Management includes medical nutrition therapy, weight management, blood glucose monitoring, and medications if needed. The table below illustrates the general recommendations for weight gain during pregnancy.

Table: Recommendation for weight gain during pregnancy

BMI	Recommended weight gain
Underweight (BMI <18)	28-40 lbs
Healthy weight (BMI 19-24)	24-35 lbs
Overweight (BMI 25-29)	15-25 lbs
Obese (BMI >30)	11-20 lbs

Treatment

Currently, insulin is the standard of care in treatment of diabetes during pregnancy. None of the insulin's are formally FDA approved however regular insulin, basal insulin Levemir, intermediate acting insulin NPH and several short acting insulin analogs like insulin aspart and lispro are considered safe to be used in pregnancy. There is not enough human data available for oral medications and other insulins to be considered safe for use during pregnancy and hence not recommended. You must talk to your doctor as soon as the pregnancy is confirmed to make the necessary medication changes. If you have Type 1 or Type 2 diabetes, you may also be on a cholesterol medication like statin or blood pressure medication like ACE inhibitors, both of which cannot be used during pregnancy and must be discontinued. Women with diabetes have to be closely monitored and must be seen as frequently as every 4 weeks or sooner.

Insulin requirement continues to increase during the second and third trimester of pregnancy, and frequent adjustment of insulin dose is needed. Staying physically active and exercising is equally important during pregnancy. The type of exercise depends on the time of pregnancy and the presence of complications. Activities like yoga, swimming, and biking are encouraged during pregnancy.

Women with diabetes are at increased risk for developing diabetic eye disease. If retinopathy is already present, a progression or worsening may be seen. A dilated diabetic eye exam is advised for all women upon confirmation of pregnancy and with each trimester.

Eating Well

Women with diabetes need to eat foods that are more nourishing and cause less elevation in blood glucose. Fresh fruits and vegetables, whole grains, and lean proteins are advised. It is strongly recommended to work with a diabetes educator or dietitian during your pregnancy. During delivery, insulin dose may need aggressive adjustment as you may not need as much insulin as before. When you start labor, insulin requirements significantly decrease. If insulin is not adjusted, glucose may drop immediately after the delivery of the baby. If your blood glucose was uncontrolled during pregnancy, your newborn baby may be at risk of hypoglycemia upon birth. As the baby has regular feedings, glucose usually returns to normal.

Breastfeeding

The American Diabetes Association strongly encourages all women with diabetes to breastfeed their babies. Breast milk provides essential nutrients to boost a baby's immune system. Breastfeeding also helps the mom to lose weight. Blood glucose may drop during breastfeeding. One may need a little snack before breastfeeding to avoid hypoglycemic reaction.

MANAGEMENT OF DIABETES AROUND MENOPAUSE

Hormonal changes associated with menopause can impact the blood glucose levels similar to that with menses. In addition to night sweats, hot flashes, and mood swings, fluctuation in blood glucose levels is common with menopause. During menopause, the levels of estrogen and progesterone drop in a woman's body. As you make less estrogen, the body becomes less sensitive to insulin and, therefore, glucose may run high despite eating the same diet as before. Menopause brings a lot of changes in a woman's body and dealing with high glucose along with menopausal symptoms may be overwhelming. Some women may experience mood swings and irritability around menopause; this can have a big impact on how they are managing their diabetes. Talk to a therapist or your healthcare provider if you feel you need help. Seeing a therapist or joining online or neighborhood support groups might also be helpful.

Yeast Infections

Yeast infections are very common in women with diabetes. Risk further increases during menopause as estrogen levels decline and the lining of the vagina changes, making it more susceptible to infections. Fungus likes to grow in the setting of high blood glucose. As more glucose is excreted in urine, it helps fungus to thrive. Most yeast infections can be treated by over-the-counter antifungal medications, but severe infections may need prescription medication.

Chapter 11

DIABETES IN MEN

ERECTILE DYSFUNCTION

Erectile dysfunction is defined as the inability to achieve an erection or maintain an erection long enough for sexual intercourse. Erectile dysfunction is a common problem in men with diabetes. More than half of the men over 50 have experienced some degree of ED also called impotency. Erectile dysfunction is associated with long-term uncontrolled diabetes. Both psychological and physical factors are involved in the development of erectile dysfunction. Diabetics have increased risk of nerve damage and blood vessel damage, both of which can have an impact on sexual performance.

Nerve damage may destroy the nerve endings signaling to the penis, whereas blood vessel damage can lead to decreased circulation, causing erectile dysfunction. Both nerve damage and blood vessel damage can be prevented by keeping blood glucose in good control. Certain medications like antidepressants, blood pressure medications, and antihistamines can also lead to erectile dysfunction.

Talking to your doctor is the best way to identify the factors contributing to erectile dysfunction and getting appropriate treatment. It may be sometimes difficult to bring up the topic for discussion. But do not hesitate to mention your concerns and symptoms to your doctor. Your doctor is a trained professional and should be comfortable to have a conversation to diagnose and treat erectile dysfunction.

Several medications are available for treatment of ED. Most of these work by improving the blood flow to the penis. It should be kept in mind that certain medications used for treatment of erectile dysfunction cannot be combined with certain other medications such as nitrates. It is important to let your doctor know about all your medications prior to starting treatment. For those who cannot take any of these medications, certain other treatments, such as using a vacuum device or a pump and penile implants and some other options, are available.

LOW TESTOSTERONE

Testosterone is the most important hormone for men. It has many functions, including sexual desire and libido. Testosterone levels slowly decline with age, but there are many other reasons for low testosterone. Men with Type 2 diabetes are twice as likely to have low testosterone levels compared to those without diabetes. Low testosterone can cause decreased libido and erectile dysfunction, weakness, low energy levels, loss of muscle mass, increase in body fat, and emotional and mental health issues. Testosterone levels can be easily checked with the help of a simple blood test. Testosterone replacement is started in those who are found to have significantly low levels after complete workup is done to exclude any problems with the pituitary glands. Testosterone replacement can be given in the form of injections, patches, gel, or implants. There is no oral testosterone formulation approved in the United states. Oral testosterone is available and approved to be used in certain countries outside the United states. Regular monitoring is required for those who are started on testosterone replacement.

Chapter 12

DIABETES IN THE ELDERLY

More than twenty-five percent of the US population aged 65 and older have diabetes. Management of diabetes in the elderly can become challenging, especially if they have uncontrolled diabetes. Older adults with diabetes are at an increased risk for developing complications. People over 65 are often excluded from clinical trials; therefore, we do not have enough evidence-based trials to come up with standards or guidelines for managing diabetes in the elderly population. This is further complicated by the physiological changes associated with aging as well as the comorbidities and functional impairment that is often present in older people. Older adults have a high risk of having heart attacks, visual impairments, kidney disease, and lower extremity amputations. Clinical characteristics of diabetes in those diagnosed before age 65 and those after 65 differ in several ways. While those diagnosed under age 65 are at high risk of complications as they age, elderly patients diagnosed with diabetes after age 65 have relatively milder diabetes, less complications, lower HbA1c, and lower likelihood of requiring insulin.

RISK OF HYPOGLYCEMIA

Risk of hypoglycemia is much more in the elderly population compared to younger population. There are several reasons for it.

1. The counter regulatory mechanisms, which help to prevent hypoglycemia and produce symptoms, are diminished in the elderly population

2. The elderly often have other comorbidities, such as heart disease or impaired kidney function, that result in decreased clearance of medication from the body

3. Appetite in the elderly can vary from day to day. Most elderly patients do not have regular meals, which can lead to hypoglycemia

4. Sometimes access to food is an issue. If the elderly do not have easy access to food, they may not eat

5. Older people can also get forgetful and end up having double dosing of the medication

6. Presence of conditions like Alzheimer's and dementia makes it worse

7. The elderly also have visual problems and may not be able to see or read the dosing correctly

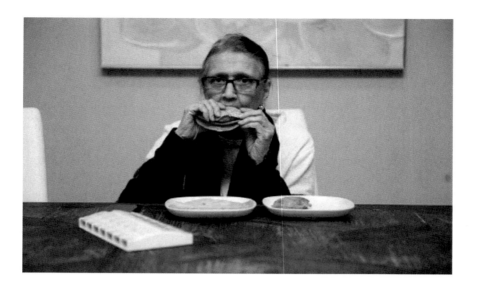

TIPS TO PREVENT HYPOGLYCEMIA IN THE ELDERLY

- Simplify the medication regimen. Talk to your doctor to see how this can be done
- Medications like glyburide or other sulfonylureas can linger on in the body for a longer time. Use of sulfonylureas is discouraged for the elderly patients, especially in those with complications
- Many alternate medications like DPP-4 inhibitors or GLP-1 agents can be safely used in the elderly with relatively lower risk of hypoglycemia
- The elderly should be encouraged to have regular meals, as skipping meals is often a common problem that leads to hypoglycemia
- The elderly with vision problems should consider using a talking glucose monitor. Talking monitors are specifically designed for patients with visual impairment. These monitors will speak aloud the glucose number in addition to the display on the screen
- Use of pill boxes is strongly encouraged in the elderly to keep track of medications
- Medication dispensing systems can also be used, which not only dispense a controlled amount of medication at a given time but also can send messages to the loved ones if the patient has taken medication or not
- The elderly are also encouraged to take other precautions of hypoglycemia such as avoiding delaying meals and keeping a glucose tablet or hard candy with them all the time for emergency treatment of hypoglycemia
- Setting up a medical alert system is also highly recommended, especially for those who live alone to get immediate help

Glucose Targets in the Elderly

Based on the American Diabetes Association guidelines, older adults who do not have cognitive issues and have normal functional status can use the same guidelines for glucose targets as normal population, which is HbA1c less than seven. For patients with cognitive problems and other comorbidities, such as heart disease, kidney disease, decreased functional status, a less stringent diabetes goal is advised. You can discuss with your doctor what HbA1c goal is appropriate for you. HbA1c, by itself, is sometimes not reliable in elderly individuals, especially if they have chronic kidney disease, which causes anemia. This can make the HbA1c falsely low. Other means of monitoring such as fasting glucose levels and Accu-check readings have to be used with these patients for monitoring and medication dose adjustments. Monitoring and glucose targets are set on an individual basis for patients with advanced complications and life expectancy less than 5 years. For these patients, it is suggested to have a more relaxed HbA1c goal preferably between 8-9.

SCREENING FOR DIABETES AND PREDIABETES IN THE ELDERLY

Based on ADA recommendations, all adults who are overweight or with risk factors and all adults over age 45 should be screened for diabetes. The benefit of screening the elderly individuals for prediabetes and diabetes depends on their functional capacity and life expectancy.

Elderly patients who have full functional capacity can get full benefit from screening for diabetes, as intervention to prevent diabetes and complications can be taken, assuming they have several years to live. However, screening for diabetes in the elderly, frail individuals with minimum functional capacity with very low life expectancy is unlikely to be beneficial.

Screening for Chronic Complications in Elderly Diabetics

Screening for certain chronic complications of diabetes is strongly advised. However, the recommendations for screening are based on evidence from studies that were mostly performed in younger individuals with long life expectancies. Elderly over age 65 who are relatively healthy with normal functional status can be screened for complications using the same guidelines as for adults. For the elderly with short life expectancy and the presence of multiple comorbidities, screening for complications is not very beneficial. However, this group should be screened for complications that would further decrease their functional status and quality of life such as foot ulcers and visual impairment.

The Elderly and Statin Medication

Statins are cholesterol lowering medications recommended in all adult diabetics between the ages of 40 to 75. This recommendation is based on the results from multiple studies that have shown to decrease cardiovascular risks and improved survival. Studies have also shown that statins continue to lower cardiovascular risk and improve survival in elderly. It is therefore advised to continue statins in the elderly except those with very limited life expectancy. Side effect profile including myalgias must be kept in mind when using statins in elderly, and lower doses are preferred.

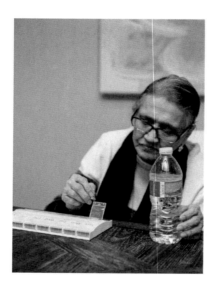

Blood Pressure

There is convincing evidence from many studies that lowering blood pressure in the elderly is associated with a decreased risk of heart attack and stroke.

Aspirin

It is recommended that as long as there are no contraindications, all individuals over 40 years of age with diabetes and cardiovascular disease must be on low dose aspirin therapy. Some elderly may need to use a proton pump inhibitor along with aspirin to decrease the risk of bleeding.

Physical Activity & Exercise for Seniors

Regular physical activity is known to prevent a variety of health conditions in the elderly like diabetes, hypertension, high cholesterol, osteoporosis, certain cancers, depression, and stroke. Exercise in the elderly is shown to improve cholesterol levels, build physical endurance, reduce falls and injuries, and enhance sleeping quality.

Adequate exercise for seniors is a minimum of 30 minutes of activity involving raising the heart rate to 75 % of maximum predicted heart rate 3-5 days a week.

Maximum Heart Rate Calculation

A person's maximum heart rate is calculated by subtracting age from 220. This is the maximum upper limit of what your heart can withstand. It is advisable to exercise within 55-85 % of the maximum heart rate. For example, the target heart rate for a 65-year-old should be 220 minus 65, which is 155 beats per minute. This is the upper limit of target heart rate for that person. Now if you want to work out at 70% of your target heart rate, you need to multiply 155 by .70 = 108. When first starting to exercise, begin with a lower target range like 60-70% for 20-30 minutes and then work your way up as tolerated. These goals can be achieved by simple exercises like walking or swimming. If chest pain, shortness of breath, chest tightness or dizziness are experienced, you must stop immediately and discuss with your doctor.

Chapter 13

DIABETES AND TRAVEL

If you are someone who loves to travel, having diabetes should not stop you from exploring the world. Traveling can disrupt your diabetes management routine, but with a little planning and some advanced preparation, you can stay healthy and enjoy your trip without any problems. Before you take the trip, you want to make sure you are healthy to travel and prepared to handle any potential emergency situation. Prior to traveling, check with your doctor well in advance if possible. Give yourself enough time before your departure so that if your doctor wants to adjust your medication you have enough time to see how it is working for you before you start your trip. If you are traveling abroad, make sure you are up to date on all the immunization you need to travel to a particular destination. Travel to certain countries may require vaccinations that are not routinely given in the United States.

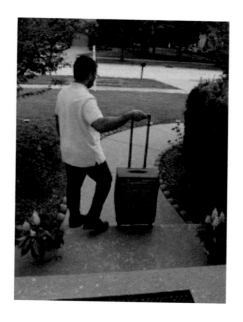

PREPARING FOR TRAVEL

Have a diabetes care kit, including information about your medical history and your list of medications and allergies, and carry it with you. This will be valuable information in case of an emergency. Have your doctor give you a letter that states all the medications, insulin, pens and needles, testing supplies, and CGM that you need to carry with you. Airport security might ask for a letter, especially if you are carrying insulin pen, syringes, or pen needles with you. Always get enough refills and carry extra medications with you, especially when traveling abroad. It will become handy if you lose your medication for some reason. If you are on an insulin pump, call your pump company for a loaner pump just in case something happens to your pump while you are abroad. Also consider taking extra pump supplies.

WEAR A MEDICAL ID BRACELET

Consider wearing a medical ID bracelet that states diabetes and other chronic conditions.

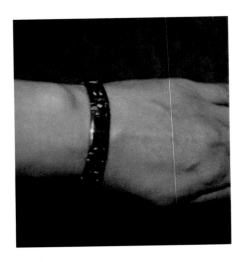

In an emergency, such as low blood sugar, it will alert the medical personnel of your diabetes. Research healthy food options at your destination so you can choose wisely. Check out restaurant menus ahead of time to see if they have a low-carb menu.

PACKING FOR YOUR TRIP

- Pack at least half of your medications in a carry-on bag so you have easy access to them; leave the other half in a checked bag. This way, if one piece of luggage is lost, you will still have some medications in your other luggage for immediate use
- If you are on insulin, it is advisable to pack it in the hand luggage, as checked-in baggage can be subject to extremes of temperature. Both very hot and very cold temperature can result in insulin losing its efficacy
- Include an extra blood glucose monitor, glucose tablets, and glucagon kit for treating low blood glucose
- Pack some healthy snacks like protein bars and peanut butter or crackers and a water bottle to carry with you in case your meal is delayed and you have to take your medications

Choosing Your Seat

When traveling by air, it is advisable to opt for an aisle seat, which will make it easier for you to get up for using the bathroom. If your blood glucose is not well controlled, you may need to use the bathroom more frequently. This will also allow you to get up and exercise by walking up and down the aisle periodically, especially during long flights.

Travel Across Time Zones

If you are traveling across time zones and need to take your insulin, remember to consider time zone changes as you fly. Remember that traveling east results in a shorter day, so you will take less insulin. On the other hand, westward travel results in a longer day so you will take more insulin.

TIPS FOR TRAVELING

- Wear comfortable clothes and shoes. You want to take extra walking shoes. Make sure you don't develop blisters from walking
- Alert those traveling with you of your diagnosis. If you are not traveling with family or close friends who know your diagnosis, make sure that you alert a co-worker, a group leader, or a person sitting next to you about your diabetes
- Check your sugars more frequently when away and take your medications regularly
- Ask your insurance company about medical coverage and treatment while abroad
- Consider getting travel insurance
- Label all of your medications to speed up getting through security
- People with diabetes are exempt from the 3.4 ounce liquid rule
- Diabetics are allowed and encouraged to keep medications, fast acting carbohydrates like juice, and gel packs to keep insulin in their hand luggage
- Pack at least half of your medications in your hand luggage
- Wear a medical ID bracelet

Chapter 14

GENETIC AND CULTURAL DISPARITIES IN DIABETES MANAGEMENT

Based on CDC data from 2017, over 30 million Americans have been diagnosed with Type 2 diabetes and another 7 million are suffering from undiagnosed diabetes. Out of the 30 million, 15.1 percent are American Indian, 12.1 percent are African American, 12.7 percent are Hispanic, 8 percent are Asian American, and 7.4 percent are Caucasian.

Scientist have linked several gene mutations to a higher risk of diabetes. Not everyone who carries a mutation has diabetes. Individually, the contribution from each gene mutation is very small. However, the risk significantly increases when combined with a host of environmental and cultural factors. Cultural factors like eating habits, food choices, religious beliefs, and lack of trust in the system has a big impact on development of diabetes in addition to the medical and environmental factors like obesity, family history, hypertension, high triglycerides, and history of gestational diabetes.

Minority groups like African Americans, Asians, Native Americans, and Hispanics bear a disproportionate burden of the diabetes epidemic. They are more likely to develop Type 2 diabetes and less likely to maintain effective control and have higher rates of complications

RISK OF DIABETES IN AFRICAN AMERICANS

When compared to non-Hispanic whites, African Americans have 77 percent higher risk of developing diabetes overall. They also have three times higher risk of developing chronic kidney disease and end stage renal disease. African Americans have 2.2 times higher risk of getting hospitalized for diabetes and two to three times higher risk of death from complications of diabetes. In one study comparing increased incidence of DKA in African American population, cessation of insulin was a major precipitating factor. Out of patients tested, 40 percent stopped insulin due to lack of means to get refills for insulin and another 25 percent stopped due to fundamental misunderstanding of the role of insulin on sick days. The remaining 35 percent did not have a specific reason. Nearly two-thirds of the cases could have been prevented if they had resources to get insulin and a better understanding of what it does. Obesity is associated with insulin resistance and a risk factor for Type 2 diabetes. Obesity is more prevalent among African Americans than White Americans, especially in African American women; it is estimated that diabetes can be attributed to abdominal obesity in 39.9 percent of African American women, compared with 24.0 percent of white American women. Additionally, physical activity is decreased in African-American women. This also contributes to their risk for diabetes. Moreover, African American children, especially girls, have a higher rate of insulin resistance than Caucasian children. In addition to the above, lack of resources and socio-economic status makes it harder for some groups to manage their diabetes effectively.

RISK OF DIABETES IN HISPANICS

Compared to non-Hispanic whites, Hispanics are 84 percent more likely to develop diabetic retinopathy and 1.7 times more likely to develop ESRD. Prevalence of diabetes in Hispanic populations increases with age and is higher in women. It has been shown to be related to the length of stay in the United States. As an ethnic group, Hispanics have high rates of diabetes. It has been observed that not all Hispanics are at equal risk for developing Type 2 diabetes. Hispanics of Mexican and Puerto Rican origin have a higher risk compared with those from other Central American or South American backgrounds.

RISK OF DIABETES IN AMERICAN INDIANS AND NATIVE AMERICANS

Risk of diabetes in American Indians and Native Americans is, by far, the highest among all racial and ethnic groups. Clinical characteristics of diabetes in this group includes obesity, insulin resistance, insulin secretory dysfunction and increased endogenous glucose production. A recent study showed a role of a specific gene mutation that is found in one in 100,000 people worldwide. In Pima Indians, the prevalence of this gene mutation is 1 in 33 people.

RISK OF DIABETES IN ASIAN AMERICANS

Asian Americans have 30 percent higher risk of diabetes compared to non-Hispanic whites. The Asian American group, by itself, is very diverse and represents 16 different ethnicities. Asians tend to develop diabetes at a lower BMI compared to their Caucasian counterparts. Asians are also at higher risk of developing gestational diabetes at a lower body weight. It is, therefore, important to consider using the BMI chart specially made for Asian population when calculating BMI for an Asian person. Among Asian Americans, 23 percent of those from India, Pakistan, and other South Asian countries have diabetes, while only 14 percent of those of Chinese, Japanese, and Korean descent do. Experts suggest that cultural traditions affecting obesity may play a role for such differences among ethnic groups.

Among the Asian sub-groups, South Asians had the highest prevalence of diabetes. South Asians are shown to have more insulin resistance and rapid decline in beta cells at a younger age compared to other Asians and Caucasians. South Asians have a unique phenotype with high waist measurements, indicating central body obesity. This is associated with a characteristic metabolic profile with high insulin levels, greater degree of insulin resistance, and high prevalence of diabetes and prediabetes.

Your health care provider may look at your BMI to determine whether you are overweight or obese. For most people, that means a BMI of 25 or greater. But for Asian Americans, who may be at risk for diabetes even at a normal weight, a BMI of 23 or greater is considered overweight

If you fall within one of the particularly high-risk subgroups, talk to your doctor or your specialist about being screened for diabetes at an earlier age. Have a discussion with your health care specialist about your family history, diet, eating habits, and physical activity.

Whatever your ethnic background, you are not destined to get diabetes, As mentioned before, a weight loss of even 5-7 percent in overweight people with prediabetes reduces the risk of progressing to Type 2 diabetes by as much as 58 percent.

Despite academic interest, participation of minorities in clinical trials is very scant. One NIH study showed most participants from ethnic groups will participate in phase one trial but leave before the start of phase 2 when actual randomization occurs. It is important that minority groups participate in clinical studies, especially drug studies so that the behavior of different medications can be studied in different ethnicities. Disparities in diabetes management occurs worldwide. It is crucial to recognize the differences in genetic makeup and cultural and environmental risk factors for diabetes in different ethnic populations and keep those factors in mind during management of diabetes.

Chapter 15

COVID-19 PANDEMIC AND DIABETES

This book is being written in the middle of the COVID-19 pandemic. It would not be complete if I did not discuss the impact of COVID-19 on people with diabetes. COVID-19 started in China around the beginning of 2020. Since then, it has spread around the world and has been declared as a pandemic by the World Health Organization. To date, over 20 million people have been infected with Covid-19 across the globe and over 730,000 people have died.

COVID-19 is a new, serious Corona virus. The Corona virus was first discovered in 1960. There are many different strains of Corona viruses. They're transmitted from animals to humans. These viruses can cause infections ranging from mild respiratory symptoms to severe life-threatening illness. The SAR-COV virus caused the acute adult respiratory distress syndrome. COVID-19 is the SAR-COV2 virus that causes respiratory illness, which, in severe cases, can cause serious infection of the lungs, leading to pneumonia, kidney failure, and even death.

Today, as COVID-19 continues to persist in several countries globally, with the death toll still rising in some countries, it's important for everyone to take the necessary precautions to help prevent infection and spread of the virus. Individuals over 60 years of age and those with preexisting medical conditions, including diabetes, are at the highest risk for complications. Based on current CDC data, 94 percent of COVID-19 deaths in U.S. had underlying medical conditions.

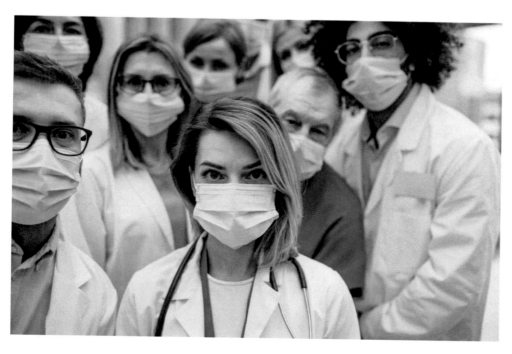

HOW IS THE VIRUS TRANSMITTED?

COVID-19 is transmitted through air droplets that are dispersed when an infected person coughs, sneezes, or talks. The virus is thought to enter the body through mucous membranes of the nose, mouth, and eyes. It can be spread through close contact with the infected person or by contact with droplets in the environment such as touching an object that has droplets and then touching your mouth, eyes, or nose.

SIGNS AND SYMPTOMS OF COVID-19 INFECTION

Symptoms may start in 3-7 days after exposure to the virus, but, in some cases, it may take up to 14 days. Therefore, a quarantine of 14 days is advised for anyone who has had potential exposure to the virus.

- Fever with or without chills
- Shortness of breath
- Chest pain
- Loss of taste and smell
- Headache
- Fatigue
- Nausea
- Vomiting
- Diarrhea
- Sore throat
- Muscle ache

HOW DOES COVID-19 IMPACT A PERSON WITH DIABETES?

At this time, scientists all over the world are still learning about Covid-19. We do not have enough data to prove that people with diabetes are at increased risk for COVID-19 infection; however, with the limited experience that we have so far, it has been observed that people with diabetes who got infected with Covid-19 have had much higher rate of complications and increased mortality compared to those who did not have diabetes. The exact mechanism by which the virus influences glucose metabolism is still unclear. Several factors could predispose diabetic patients to infections. These include:

- Genetic susceptibility to infection
- Altered cellular immune defenses
- Local factors including poor blood supply and nerve damage

- Alterations in metabolism
- Depressed antioxidant systems and humoral immunity in diabetes

Effect of Hyperglycemia on Immune Response

Hyperglycemia affects several aspects of cellular immune function like chemotaxis, adherence, phagocytosis, and intracellular killing. Anaerobic conditions in the tissue that are created by vascular compromise and inflammatory response further impair the immune response.

Risk of Lung Infection in Diabetes

Diabetics are also at an increased risk for lung infection. High blood glucose is thought to damage the blood vessels in the lungs the same way as it damages the blood vessels in other organs. Damage to lung tissue results in diminished diffusion of oxygen. The extent of the changes in lung tissue seems to depend on the level of glycemic control.

Diabetics also are susceptible to pulmonary infections because of an increased risk of aspiration secondary to gastroparesis, diminished cough reflex, and disordered sleep patterns. It has also been reported that diabetics may be more likely to have recurrent pneumonia.

When people with uncontrolled glucose develop a COVID-19 infection, it can be harder to treat due to fluctuations in blood glucose levels and presence of complications. This is due to two reasons:

1. The immune system in diabetics is compromised, making it harder to fight the infection and recovery may take longer
2. The virus may thrive in an environment of elevated blood glucose

DOES COVID-19 CAUSE DIABETES?

Some scientist suggests a dual relationship between COVID-19 and diabetes. They postulate that COVID-19 may trigger changes in glucose metabolism by causing damage to the pancreas resulting in worsening of preexisting diabetes and development of new diabetes. However, there is no evidence to prove this hypothesis and more research is needed to unfold this.

RISK OF DIABETIC KETOACIDOSIS WITH COVID-19

It has been observed that diabetics have an increased risk of developing diabetic ketoacidosis when infected with COVID-19, especially those with uncontrolled diabetes. Those who did develop DKA suffered from more complications with prolonged recovery times.

WHAT PRECAUTIONS SHOULD A DIABETIC TAKE?

Because people with diabetes may also have other comorbidities, such as organ failure and Cardiovascular Disease, it is imperative that they follow specific COVID-19 precautions and prevention guidelines from the CDC and WHO along with the instructions provided by their endocrinologist or health care provider.

- Diabetics are advised to monitor glucose frequently so fluctuations can be detected early and treated
- Diabetics should also take prescribed medications regularly, have ample supply of diabetes medications, and call their provider for adjustment in medication if glucose is running high
- They must also watch their diet carefully, stay hydrated, and try to be physically active
- People are advised to avoid using any alternative medicine for prevention of COVID-19 as there is none available
- They must cover their nose and mouth with mask at all times when in public as recommended by local authorities
- They must maintain social distancing at least 6 feet distance from another person
- They must make every possible effort to avoid contact with a potentially exposed or infected person
- They must wash hands frequently with soap and warm water
- They must avoid unnecessary travel, public transportation, or large gatherings

WHAT TO DO IF SOMEONE IS SICK WITH COVID-19 IN YOUR HOME?

- Person must stay in a separate room if possible
- Person must avoid close contact with other family members
- Household contacts who are already exposed must quarantine for 14 days to avoid further spread of the virus
- Person must not share utensils and all surfaces must be cleaned regularly
- Only one family member should take care of the sick person to avoid minimal exposure of the rest of the family members
- Elderly populations and those with long-term diabetes or advanced diabetic complications are particularly at risk of early death, and may require specific precautions to avoid infection

TREATMENT

At present, there is no vaccine or antiviral treatment available for COVID-19. The most effective treatment currently is supportive treatment. Several medications have been tried but none have proven to be curative.

Hydroxychloroquine

Was initially used in the treatment with the idea of reducing mortality; however, currently available data have shown that it does not reduce mortality in hospitalized patients and, instead, was associated with life-threatening side effects.

Antiviral Treatment

Several other antiviral treatments have also been tried in treating COVID-19, but none have proven to be effective enough to completely treat COVID-19 infection.

Remdesivir an antiviral RNA polymerase inhibitor has been shown to shorten the length of hospital stays in Covid patients.

Dexamethasone

This is a corticosteroid that has been used for years as a lifesaving drug in critically ill patients. It is the first medication that has been shown to save lives in COVID-19 patients. However, it is only modestly effective in outside ICU setting. Several clinical trials are being done currently to study the role and effectiveness of dexamethasone for treatment of COVID-19 infection.

Interferon

There is also some data on use of inhaled interferon lowering the risk of severe infection and increased likelihood of recovering from COVID-19 infection.

COVID-19 Vaccine

Scientist all over the world are putting their heads together to create a vaccine for corona virus. No vaccine is 100 percent effective but a vaccine would provide some protection by training people's immune system to fight the virus. A vaccine would normally take years to develop. Researchers are trying to get the same amount of work done in few months. Most researchers think a vaccine will be available soon. Let us keep our fingers crossed and be optimistic. The world has seen five worse pandemics end. This shall pass too.

About the Author

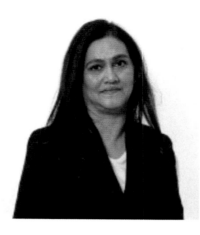

Dr. Nuzhat Chalisa is a clinical Endocrinologist practicing in Chicago for the past 20 years. Dr. Chalisa completed residency training in Internal medicine at Loyola University Medical Center in Chicago. She did fellowship in Endocrinology Diabetes and Metabolism & Nutrition at the Rosalind Franklin University of Health Sciences in Chicago IL. She is a fellow of American College of Endocrinology.

Dr. Chalisa's primary interest has been in the area of diabetes and obesity. Her experience crosses between research and clinical practice. Outside of clinical practice she has keen interest in community work and teaching. Some of her initial research was on age-related cognitive decline in diabetics and continuous glucose monitoring. Currently, she has been working on recognizing and minimizing racial and ethnic disparities in diabetes management. Dr. Chalisa has published several articles on diabetes and related topics. She has been a frequent guest speaker in several national and international diabetes and obesity conferences.

Dr. Chalisa currently serves as the Communications Director for ADA's Clinical Centers and Program Interest Group Leadership Team.

Dr. Chalisa is also the founder and president of a diabetes nonprofit organization called "Kisat Diabetes Organization," the main mission of which is to prevent diabetes complications through early screening and education. She is actively involved with multiple community awareness programs in the Chicago area.

Visit her website at: nuzhatchalisamd.com

Can You Help?

Thank You For Reading My Book!

I would really appreciate your feedback, and would love hear what you have to say.

I need your input to make the next version of this book and my future books better.

Please leave me an honest review on Amazon letting me know what you thought of the book.

Thanks so much!

Nuzhat Chalisa MD, FACE

Made in the USA
Columbia, SC
27 July 2021